Antonio SANDU

THE MEDICALIZATION OF SOCIAL LIFE

Anxiety and frustration in times of pandemics

2025

LUMEN

în elita editurilor românești

THE MEDICALIZATION OF SOCIAL LIFE
Anxiety and frustration in times of pandemics
Antonio SANDU

redactia@edituralumen.net
www.edituralumen.ro

Descrierea CIP a Bibliotecii Naţionale a României
SANDU, ANTONIO
The medicalization of social life : anxiety and frustration in times of pandemics / Antonio Sandu. - Iaşi : Lumen, 2025
Conţine bibliografie
ISBN 978-973-166-647-1

316

Table of contents

Introduction

Anxiety is defined as a state of unease, tense anticipation, accompanied by palpitations and difficulty breathing, often encountered in nervous disorders (Romanian Academy, 2009). Another definition, derived from NODEX (2002), describes anxiety as a pathological state of restlessness, an undetermined fear, frequently accompanied by physiological disturbances.

Frustration, according to the same dictionary, has multiple connotations, including: "depriving someone of a rightful entitlement", also understood as a loss, deprivation of satisfaction - often of a sexual nature -, deception; disappointment, or the state of an individual who, due to an obstacle or inhibition, cannot fulfill a desire or satisfy a pleasure.

The Covid-19 pandemic has led to the restriction of entire societies, with or without genuine public health expertise justification, imposing limitations on freedom of movement, mandating specific social behaviors - such as social distancing, mask-wearing, and the shift of much public activity to the online environment (virtualization of social space), among others.

A series of studies conducted during the first wave of the Coronavirus pandemic, when almost all countries worldwide were in a state of lockdown and quarantine, demonstrate that the spread of the SARS-COV-2 virus has had a significant impact on populations across various communities. Consequently, Nader Salari and colleagues (Salari et al., 2020) argue that psychological measures should be implemented during the pandemic to improve the mental health of the population, particularly for vulnerable groups. As the effects of the pandemic, especially on mental/psychological and psychosocial health, continue to manifest even after five years, the results of research on anxiety and frustration experienced by the population during the pandemic can be beneficial both theoretically and pragmatically for those involved in constructing public health policies, as well as for clinical psychologists or those providing psychotherapy and psychological/ philosophical counseling to individuals affected by the pandemic.

Although now, more than a year after the emergence of the first SARS-COV-2 infection cases, we are facing successive waves of this pandemic - with shorter or longer, intermittent periods of local lockdowns, as well as other phenomena such as vaccine hesitancy, which can be attributed to the frustration accumulated during the March-June 2020 period of the first major lockdown following the outbreak of the pandemic.

The effect of the psychological crisis is considered by Nader and colleagues to be more pronounced in patients in the early stages of mental disorders, potentially leading to psychological changes, including at a pathological level. The most probable pathologies are those determined by fear, anxiety, depression, or insecurity (Zhang et al., 2020), pathologies which are accentuating the phenomenon of medicalization of social life.

The research that forms the subject of this study was conducted during the pandemic period itself, based on interviews with 103 individuals, and aimed to highlight the phenomena of anxiety and anguish caused by the restrictions imposed during the pandemic, as well as the dimensions of the medicalization of social life generated by this pandemic. Partial results of the research have been previously published in scientific journals, in works that will be appropriately cited throughout this volume and duly mentioned in its bibliography. However, they have never been compiled into a standalone volume that provides the reader with a complex and comprehensive picture of the phenomenon as it was experienced, particularly by individuals in the North-Eastern region of Romania directly affected by the lockdown or the pandemic.

As this is essentially research conducted during March-May 2020, we will occasionally preserve the tone of the responses and their dynamics, expressed in the present tense, to familiarize the reader with the emotional state of the respondents and their discursive perspective from the very moment of the lockdown. These elements contributed decisively to the social construction of the pandemic and to the understanding, from a social-constructionist perspective, of the phenomenon of medicalization of social life, as it was accentuated by/during the pandemic period.

Cap. I. Theoretical Perspectives on Anxiety and Frustration in the Context of Covid-19 Pandemics

In the context of the pandemic triggered by the SARS-COV-2 virus, a series of measures were implemented, including the quarantine of certain localities, global population lockdowns, mandatory social distancing and mask-wearing, and limited access to health services - other than those for the care of Covid patients. In this context, the emergence of individual behaviors generated by fear of health deterioration and possible death is foreseeable. Additionally, the feeling of helplessness and the required stereotypical social behaviors (Salari et al., 2020) - including social distancing - can, in the opinion of consulted psychologists, generate a large-scale psychological crisis that may represent a real threat to public mental health (Xiang et al., 2020).

I.1. Anxiety – operational definitions and ethiology

According to the Encyclopaedia Britannica (2021), *anxiety* represents a feeling of strong apprehension, fear, or unease, often without a clear justification. *Anxiety* is distinguished from *fear* precisely by this vague character of the sensation that appears in response to an indistinct danger (sometimes only intuited), while the latter state occurs in response to a clear and evident danger that affects the person's physical safety. Anxiety is a subjective response to an internal emotional conflict, the causes of which may not be evident to the person experiencing the state of anxiety. When the state of anxiety is intense - being recurrent or chronic and cannot be justified as representing a response to stressful stimuli from everyday life - it is considered an *emotional disorder*.

Anxiety Disorder is one of the most widespread pathologies (Bystritsky, 2013) affecting the mental health of populations worldwide. Kessler and colleagues (Kessler et al., 1994) show that this type of disorder affected 13.3% of the U.S. population in 2013, with the percentage increasing compared to previous years. Anxiety disorders constitute the most significant subgroup of mental illnesses that occur globally, although they are predominantly studied in developed countries. Anxiety disorders are considered responsible for decreased productivity in individuals suffering from this type of illness, as well as for increased morbidity and mortality rates (Leon et al.,

1995) among these individuals, or the incidence of alcohol and substance abuse (Bystritsky, 2013).

The subgroup of mental illnesses represented by anxiety disorders encompasses a series of syndromes, among which DSM-5 (The Diagnostic and Statistical Manual of Mental Disorders, Fifth Edition) (APA, 2013) emphasizes *Generalized Anxiety Disorder* (Reynolds, 2013). This disorder involves excessive anxiety and worry that persists for a period of at least 6 months.

In DSM-4, anxiety disorders included: *Panic Disorder* with or without agoraphobia, social phobia, specific phobias towards animals, environment, injections, or various situations, *Post-Traumatic Stress Disorder*, *Acute Stress Disorder*, *Obsessive-Compulsive Disorder*, and other anxiety disorders. DSM-5 redefines anxiety disorders, removing Post-Traumatic Stress Disorder and Obsessive-Compulsive Disorder from this category, reclassifying them as separate classes of mental disorders (Bystritsky, 2013).

I.2. Social Anxiety

The same manual mentioned above (APA, 2013) defines *Social Anxiety Disorder* as a condition in which social interactions generate a state of constant stress for the subject, leading them either to avoid frequent social interactions and contact or to experience these interactions in a painful manner due to a disproportionate fear of the actual social context (Reynolds, 2013). The fundamental anguish, which is often the foundation of social phobias, is the fear of others' judgment. It involves the person's fear that they will not be able to cope adequately in the given situation, subsequently being negatively labeled by others.

Prior to the emergence of DSM-5, which constructs an entire class of anxiety disorders, *Social Anxiety Disorder* was known as *Social Phobia*, thus being reclassified as a standalone disorder (Heimberg, 2014).

Usually, the person suffering from social anxiety recognizes that their fear is irrational; nevertheless, they continue to exhibit symptoms of anxiety (sweating, lump in the throat, tics, stuttering) before and during a situation that requires them to perform a social role (Medicover, 2021).

The symptoms of social anxiety and, concurrently, its diagnostic criteria are:

- Fear or anxiety about social contexts in which the person feels observed and potentially evaluated; for adults, such situations may include a first date, a job interview, an oral presentation, etc.;
- Typically, individuals experience a state of fear of social rejection;
- Social interactions generally cause them stress;
- Social interactions are generally avoided or endured with difficulty;
- Fear and anxiety occur as reactions to social situations or contexts lasting 6 months or more;
- Fear and anguish cause the individual a state of discomfort, diminishing their functionality in one or more areas, such as interpersonal relationships or professional activity;

- Fear and anxiety cannot be attributed to concrete medical causes, substance abuse, or adverse reactions to certain medications, nor do they appear as symptoms associated with other mental disorders;
- In the presence of another mental disorder, fear and anxiety appear to be uncorrelated or disproportionate to the symptoms of that medical condition; therefore, the symptoms cannot be classified under the diagnosis of Social Anxiety Disorder.

Compared to anxiety disorders in general, which had a prevalence of 13.3% in the United States in 2013, social anxiety had a prevalence of only 7% in the same year in the same country (Reynolds, 2013).

Social anxiety can manifest as withdrawal from the social environment and isolation, often accompanied by depression and *Body Dysmorphic Disorder* (BDD). However, the same symptoms of withdrawal and social isolation can be associated with other disorders, such as *Delusional Disorder*, *Autism spectrum disorders*, or *personality disorders* (Porter, n.d.).

According to DSM-5 (APA, 2013), the diagnosis of social anxiety must take into account the cultural component of personality and how individuals construct the rationality of their fears based on the dominant cultural experience in their society. As per the aforementioned manual, culture refers to the system of knowledge, concepts, rules, and practices learned and transmitted transgenerationally, including language, religion, spirituality, family structures, life cycle stages, rituals and customs, and moral and legal systems. In contemporary society, individuals are exposed to multiple cultures, which they use in constructing their own identity and to build the meaning of their own experience.

As such, cultural differences can be discovered in the rationalization of fear - a key element in diagnosing anxiety disorders - differences that must be taken into account when discussing social anxiety. It is worth noting that DSM-5 introduces the concept of *Cultural Syndrome*, with significant influences regarding anxiety. As an example of a cultural syndrome, Heimberg and colleagues (Heimberg et al., 2014) cite the *Taijin Kyofusho* (TKS) syndrome, encountered in subjects belonging to Japanese or Korean cultures, which is based on the subject's concern not to make gestures or actions that would offend or embarrass others. In contrast, the authors mention that subjects from Western cultures generally manifest social anxiety in the form of fear of entering or being put in embarrassing situations themselves.

Both forms of social anxiety manifestation can currently be encountered - in American patients on whom the studies cited by DSM-5 were conducted - due to cultural contamination and the interculturality of postmodern society.

Another cultural difference is related to individualism versus collectivism. In collectivist cultures, social harmony constitutes a priority, while the individual occupies a peripheral place in terms of societal development. In individualistic cultures, the person holds a central position, and community harmony is, at best, a secondary concern of the individual, subordinated to concerns for personal well-being and self-affirmation. Despite the different symptomatology generated by the cultural context, the common element is given by the discrepancy between the social expectations perceived by the individual and their self-perception, according to which the individual considers themselves capable or not of fulfilling social expectations or performing in their social role, in accordance with the constructs of the society to which they belong.

Therefore, social anxiety creates a disorder that puts the individual in a position of suffering - acute or chronic - and performative inefficiency of the tasks or roles they have to fulfill. In our opinion, social anxiety is socially constructed through mechanisms of interpretative drift of the significance of role performance, in the context of appropriating the cultural values of the society to which the individual belongs and/or anticipatory resocialization in different cultural contexts.

I.3. Risc Society and Medicalization of Social Life

As such socially constructed maladies - like social anxiety - acquire significant incidence from a public health perspective, and society reacts by accepting the pathological, we begin to speak of a profoundly medicalized society. The idea of a medicalized society is often connected with that of a risk society when medical risks are involved that society is partially incapable of managing otherwise than by emphasizing the pathologization of any modified psychological or social conditions, in order not to "miss" the objective of sustainable social development which consists of providing specialized care to all those presumed to need it.

"The medicalization of society represents, practically, the effect of the 'risk society' (Williams & Calnan, 1996), of the fact that society more easily becomes aware of the various risks by which individuals feel threatened. Sometimes it goes as far as the idea of 'medicalization of the human condition', which is nothing more than a *treatable disorder*." (Conrad, 2007). The medicalization of social life, as we understand it, is "an excessive use of instruments originally from the medical sphere, but poorly or unscientifically adapted to everyday life, which mark our daily lives." (Sandu, 2020).

We consider that a distinction must be made between real mental illness and existential anguish. The idea of madness in everyday life, formulated by Freud (2010), includes various disorders, from psychosis to neurosis, including everyday neurotic manifestations, with Freud concluding that, in fact, all individuals manifest some form of neurosis. While Freud privileged a therapeutic line based on psychoanalysis as a form of psychotherapy (Freud, 2010), which includes dream analysis, various oneiric creations, the person's creative acts, interactions between pseudo-therapists and patients, and life stories, under the influence of medicalization and pharmacological development, any aspect related to a so-called mental imbalance or state of social maladjustment or vulnerability came to be treated with medication. The pharmacological suppression of distressing states with neurotic potential leads to the loss of fundamental properties of human consciousness related to self-reflection, the capacity for self-knowledge, including the inherent loss of an essential component of quality of life, related to a "philosophical" lifestyle based on self-examination and reflection on ourselves. "Whether such a lifestyle based on self-knowledge and self-examination is important or not - each person is called to answer for themselves."(Sandu, 2020).

The term "risk society" was proposed by Ulrich Beck (1992), who extends the traditional concept of risk, understood as the sum of the probability of an adverse event occurring and the magnitude of its consequences, to include the subjective perception of risk - which appears in the intersubjective communication of risk - as well as the social experience of living in a risky environment. Ultimately, risk society theorists assert that not only health and the environment are in danger, but also fundamental sociopolitical values: freedom, equality, justice, respect for individual rights and democracy (Ekberg, 2007).

Current society self-defines as a "post" society: post-industrial, post-truth society, a society in post-history, but also post-secular society, the dawn of post-humanity; all these phrases define, in one form or another, postmodern society.

Postmodern society uses deconstruction as a pretext to distance itself from both the traditional and the modern - whether we're talking about social institutions (such as family), religious elements (including elements of a new religiosity), or the rise of secular humanism.

Postmodern society is balanced, at the level of social existence, by a transmodern society, which aims to be a knowledge society, fundamentally transforming the mode of production from tangible goods and services to intangible goods and services - mere noetic constructs.

The society we live in is not one where the risks citizens are subjected to are much greater than in previous societies along the historical timeline, but they are merely different and much more consciously recognized, due to consumerism and the increased quality of life, which individuals expect to be accompanied by a minimization of everyday life risks.

Life expectancy is higher than in past historical epochs, methods of treating diseases are more effective, and citizens have access to better-organized services.

Managing the risk society is more difficult to achieve because the population is more clearly and evidently aware of the risks to which it is exposed.

I.4. Management of Trust in the Risk Society

In the case of the pandemic under discussion, one of the most important ethical issues is the social construction of trust in the healthcare system as a whole. This is not necessarily a new issue, but the crisis caused by Covid-19 underscores the need for trust in the measures taken by the medical system, including those restricting individual autonomy and fundamental freedoms.

Essentially, it is about trust in public health, which suddenly seems to become imperialistic, partially subordinating public policy systems at both state and supra-state levels.

Trust in public institutions and, along with it, trust in the healthcare and public health systems, is minimized due to the exaggerated number of false news and partial information that appears, from those referring to the synthetic origin of the Coronavirus to those referring to the fact that we are in a situation of hybrid warfare between globalism and nationalism, between transnational corporations and globalizing vectors, be they state or supra-state, corporatist, and nation-states, on the other hand, which act somewhat independently, presumably in the interest of their own citizens.

The lack of trust is accentuated by the competition for medical resources, equipment, and medical personnel, a competition that takes place behind the collaboration between states or even to its detriment, in a context where there is a crisis of authorities regarding social communication, a distrust of real communication between states.

I.5. Medicalizatin of Social Life

The Covid-19 pandemic has led to the restriction of entire societies, with or without genuine grounds in terms of public health expertise, imposing limitations on freedom of movement, mandating specific social behaviors - such as social distancing, mask-wearing, and the shift of much public activity to the online environment (virtualization of social space), among others.

The medicalization of social life brings with it a lifestyle based on sometimes exaggerated concern for health conditions, increased consumption of pharmacological products or, conversely, natural products that are presumed to have an almost miraculous effect in maintaining health.

We speak of healthy lifestyles, organic lifestyles, and so on, which are imposed on us precisely by the fear of losing our comfort and health, in a context where we are aware of the risks to which we are exposed due to various elements of daily life.

The medicalization of social life, as we understand it, is an excessive use of instruments originally from the medical sphere, but poorly or unscientifically adapted to everyday life, which mark our daily existence.

I.6. Pandemics and Social Fear

Throughout history, social fear has been directed towards various manifestations of subjective otherness, such as the supernatural (divine, demonic, or magical), the *foreigner* in the literal sense (the one belonging to another culture, religion, civilization, or perceived to have divergent interests from those of one's own community), the *dysmorphic* (the one who does not share the same morphic characteristics as the fearful individual, those of another race, the "sick" or even the imagined dysmorphic: pygmies, giants, etc.).

The fear of disease and the sick polarizes social imagination, being generated by a threat that can take on an immediate character - a propagating pandemic - and about which there is a cultural memory that includes devastating experiences for the community. The plague is such an example, being a disease that terrified Europe for centuries. Alongside the plague, history has recorded the devastating effects of typhoid fever pandemics, Spanish flu, as well as recent threats of avian flu, swine flu pandemics, and their possible mutations.

Jean Delumeau, in his volume *Frica în Occident* [Fear in the West] (Delumeau, 2021) analyzes, from a historical and anthropological perspective, collective behaviors during the plague that affected Europe between 1348 and 1720. From the 14th century until the 16th century, Delumeau tells us, the plague appeared every year in one part or another of Western Europe. The chroniclers of the time called the successive appearances of the disease "first plague," "second plague," ... "sixth plague," in a manner somewhat similar to how contemporary epidemiologists count the waves of the current Covid pandemic. The historical experience of pandemics, which Delumeau speaks about, involves the disappearance of up to 40% of the population of a significant European community in a single such wave of the plague pandemic.

Therefore, the collective memory and, especially, the historiographical memory of humanity has generated a feeling of strong negative emotion - especially panic - in the early stages of the spread of the Covid-19 pandemic in China, in Europe, and then worldwide.

The cited author shows that, during the plague period, there was a state of nervousness and fear that engulfed the entire Europe (Delumeau, 2021). Boccaccio, in his book "The Decameron," states that "a multitude of sick people were so little helped, and even, because of the horror they inspired in healthy people, left prey to such cruel misery, that we can reasonably estimate at more than 100,000 the number of those who lost their lives within the city walls." (Boccaccio, 2003). Even if the figures mentioned by Boccaccio for Florence were exaggerated, historical data indeed show a mortality rate between 35%-45% in major European cities during that period, with figures of up to 60% of the population in certain cities, such as Hamburg and Bremen in Germany, being recorded by historians of the time (Delumeau, 2021).

The exceptionally long period of the plague pandemic and the devastating violence of its waves generated a social fear of pandemics. The emergence of pandemics was attributed to the will of the Divine, divine punishment, ominous astral conjunctions, or "putrid emanations from the soil or subsoil."

(Delumeau, 2021). The miasma theory led to people tasked with collecting corpses being protected with bird-beak-shaped masks - hence the term "undertakers" for people working in the funeral industry. The image of people wearing masks, as well as the isolation units from the early period of the Covid-19 pandemic, resonated in the collective mindset with the image of plague doctors from the plague period, about which the population had no direct collective memory, but an indirect one, through literary and historical evocations - often exaggerated in terms of the apocalyptic dimensions of the pandemic.

Historical works on the plague emphasized the social transmission of the pandemic from individual to individual, an element of similarity with the current pandemic, in which, among the measures taken, was social isolation or quarantine, a measure introduced for the first time for plague prevention. Epidemiologists consulted by Delumeau consider that the main agent of plague transmission was the flea, which transmitted the disease from the infected person or the deceased to the healthy one, indeed being a community transmission, but which would not have required protective measures such as wearing beak-shaped masks or quarantine, but rather hygiene and pest control measures - generally unknown at that time.

The evocation in mass media of images from past pandemics was capable of increasing the level of panic and anxiety among the population, especially in the early stages of the Covid-19 pandemic, when neither the mortality rate nor the incidence of infection per thousand inhabitants were known. In the collective mindset - medieval and modern - the plague was correlated with two other scourges, famine and war, which combined their destructive power with that of epidemics. Not coincidentally, the Covid-19 pandemic was more or less officially associated with biological weapons, with statements from the U.S. President at that time accusing China of producing biological weapons. Panic regarding food shortages manifested in the first months of the Covid-19 pandemic but was quickly neutralized by authorities' measures to over-supply food stores.

The association of the pandemic with divine wrath generates a sense of guilt, which amplifies the state of anxiety in the population, with individuals experiencing a feeling of culpability for the divine punishment befalling the community, which could be determined by their own sins as well. In the current pandemic, lockdown measures also targeted the closure of religious activities, aspects that generated sporadic dissatisfaction, which were quickly resolved by official communications and the dialogue that church institutions of most religious denominations had with both the state and the faithful.

A significant difference between the pandemic that is the subject of our work and the plague described by Jean Delumeau is the mortality level, but this level could not be known in the early period of the Covid-19 pandemic, when reports from China, Italy, or Spain highlighted a significant number of cases that exceeded the capacity of health systems to provide patient care, and mortality was estimated to be high. Uncertainty and ambivalent communication could provide sufficient grounds for panic and anguish among the population, especially those who informed themselves from alternative media sources, where the infodemic phenomenon - an epidemic of false information and news - was extremely present and difficult for authorities to counteract.

I.7. Covid 19 pandemic - an instance of social construction of the medicalization of social life

In the context of the historical evolution of global epidemiological phenomena, a pandemic distinguishes itself as a pathological manifestation of international scope, characterized by the accelerated dissemination of an infectious agent across multiple geographical regions. This phenomenon transcends the conceptual boundaries of a mere epidemic, presenting profound implications for social and economic structures on a global scale. The emergence of a pandemic is contingent upon the appearance of a novel pathogenic agent, against which the human population lacks pre-existing immune mechanisms, thus facilitating rapid and extensive human-to-human transmission.

The defining attributes of a pandemic include the capacity for sustained transmission within human communities, significant pathogenic potential, and substantial impact on healthcare systems and society as a whole. In this context, the World Health

Organization (WHO) assumes a crucial role in identifying, declaring, and monitoring pandemic phenomena, coordinating international efforts in crisis response and management (WHO, 2001).

The consequences of a pandemic extend beyond the realm of public health, profoundly affecting global economic structures, the dynamics of social relations, and international political stability. Effectively addressing such a crisis requires intense transnational collaboration, implementation of rigorous public health measures such as social isolation and quarantine, as well as acceleration of research and development processes in the therapeutic and active immunization domains.

Historical experiences, such as the 1918 Spanish flu pandemic or the recent health crisis generated by COVID-19, have highlighted the profound and multidimensional impact of pandemics on human civilization. These events have underscored the imperative of developing efficient systems for preparedness and rapid response to global epidemiological threats, emphasizing the need for a proactive and coordinated approach at the international level in managing emerging health risks.

In the context of the health crisis generated by the COVID-19 pandemic, authorities were compelled to implement a complex set of measures aimed at counteracting the spread of the SARS-CoV-2 virus and safeguarding public health. These interventions covered a wide spectrum of actions, from restricting mobility and imposing social distancing to elaborate strategies for testing, contact tracing, and subsequently, active immunization campaigns. The defining characteristic of these measures was their dynamic and adaptable nature, evolving in accordance with the progress of scientific knowledge about the pathogen, the epidemiological dynamics, and the capacity of health systems to manage increasing pressure.

In Romania, similar to other states, the response to the pandemic involved a stratified approach, encompassing decisions at the national level and specific measures implemented locally. The municipality of Suceava, which became an epicenter of the pandemic in its incipient phases, offers an example of how local authorities managed the crisis situation, adapting and intensifying general measures to the specific context of the community.

At the national level, Romania instituted a state of emergency in March 2020, followed by a state of alert, thus creating the necessary legal framework for implementing restrictions and public health measures. Significant interventions included imposing social distancing, mandatory wearing of protective masks, restricting circulation, implementing quarantine and isolation measures, suspending physical educational activities and transitioning to online learning, as well as limiting public events and gatherings.

Concurrently, testing efforts were intensified, and systems for tracing contacts of infected persons were implemented. The national vaccination campaign, initiated at the end of 2020, represented a decisive intervention in combating the pandemic. In parallel, economic support measures for employees and employers were adopted, including technical unemployment schemes.

At the level of Suceava Municipality, which experienced a particularly severe epidemiological situation in the first phase of the pandemic, specific and more restrictive measures were implemented. These included total quarantine of the city and surrounding localities, militarization of the county hospital, intensification of public space disinfection actions, organization of mass testing campaigns, and imposition of additional local restrictions based on the incidence rate.

Local authorities conducted intensive public information campaigns, adapted public services to the pandemic context through the implementation of online systems, organized support actions for vulnerable persons, and closely coordinated crisis management with national authorities. With the launch of the national vaccination campaign, the municipality organized immunization centers and actively promoted vaccination among the population.

These measures, both at national and local levels, underwent continuous evolution throughout the pandemic, being adjusted according to the epidemiological dynamics and new available information regarding the virus and methods to combat it. The experience of Suceava Municipality, especially in the initial stages of the pandemic, constituted a significant case study for managing health crises at the local level in Romania, offering valuable lessons for addressing similar situations in the future.

I.8. The concept of medicalization of social life

The concept of medicalization of social life represents a phenomenon that has gained increasing significance in the social sciences, particularly in the fields of medical sociology and medical anthropology. This theoretical construct refers to the process by which aspects of human existence, previously considered non-medical, are redefined and approached through the lens of the medical paradigm, being conceptualized in terms of pathologies or disorders. Medicalization implies an extension of modern medicine's jurisdiction beyond its traditional spheres, encompassing dimensions of daily life and human experience that were, in the past, perceived as within the limits of normality or naturalness.

Sociologists such as Peter Conrad (2007) have highlighted a pronounced tendency to interpret and manage social issues through a medical perspective. This approach has its roots in the broader critique of medicine's role in society, being significantly influenced by Michel Foucault's works on biopolitics and mechanisms of social control exercised through medical discourses and practices (Foucault, 2010).

Among the defining elements of the medicalization process are the redefinition of social problems as medical in nature, the expansion of diagnostic categories, the proliferation of medical language in public discourse, and the increased dependence on medical expertise and interventions.

This phenomenon manifests in multiple domains of social life, from the interpretation of natural processes such as aging or birth, to the approach to behavioral or emotional aspects such as sadness or hyperactivity.

Medicalization presents profound implications at both individual and societal levels. On one hand, it can lead to more effective recognition and addressing of previously neglected conditions. On the other hand, it can generate undesired effects such as the pathologization of normal human experience, excessive dependence on medical interventions, neglect of socio-economic and political factors in the etiology of health problems, and the potential stigmatization of individuals.

The phenomenon of medicalization has generated significant debates in the sphere of bioethics and medical sociology. Critics of this process argue that medicalization can erode individual autonomy, ignore cultural diversity in conceptualizing health and illness, and serve corporate interests to the detriment of public health. In contrast, supporters of medicalization emphasize its potential to improve quality of life, reduce stigma associated with certain behaviors or conditions, and stimulate innovation in the medical field.

In the context of administrative sciences, particularly in the field of public health, the analysis of the medicalization process offers a critical perspective on how contemporary society defines and approaches the concepts of health, illness, and normality. For researchers in the social sciences, a nuanced understanding of this phenomenon is essential for evaluating the implications of the expansion of the medical domain in social life and for developing balanced approaches that reconcile the benefits and risks associated with this process in the evolution of modern society.

I.9. The concept of mental health

The concept of mental health represents an essential component of individual and collective well-being, constituting a construct that has undergone significant evolution in recent decades. In the context of social sciences, the comprehension and approach to mental health are fundamental for developing effective policies and practices in the fields of public health, education, and social assistance.

The World Health Organization conceptualizes mental health as a state of well-being in which the individual actualizes their own potential, can manage daily stress, can function productively and fruitfully, and is capable of contributing to their community. This definition emphasizes that mental health transcends the mere absence of psychological pathologies, encompassing the presence of positive attributes as well (WHO, 2001).

Components of mental health include emotional, psychological, and social well-being, resilience, and optimal cognitive functioning. Factors influencing mental health are diverse, encompassing biological, psychological, social, and environmental aspects.

Within social sciences, mental health occupies a central position, influencing individuals' capacity to effectively participate in society, maintain healthy interpersonal relationships, and contribute to community development. Numerous social issues, such as poverty, criminality, and inequality, present close connections with mental health.

Contemporary approaches to studying mental health include the biopsychosocial model (Dorofte, 1997), which integrates biological, psychological, and social factors; positive psychology (Dorofte, 1991), which focuses on developing resilience and strengths; social neurosciences, which explore interactions between neural, psychological, and social processes; as well as cultural approaches, which recognize the importance of cultural context in defining and managing mental health.

Current challenges in the field of mental health aim at improving accessibility to specialized services, integrating mental health into primary care, exploring the potential offered by e-health and m-health technologies, as well as emphasizing proactive strategies for prevention and early intervention.

The concept of mental health proves to be fundamental within social sciences, offering a relevant perspective on human behavior, social interactions, and the functioning of society as a whole. As our understanding evolves, it is imperative to continue integrating knowledge from various disciplines to address the complexity of mental health and its multidimensional impact on individuals and communities.

I.10. Relevant theories in the study of mental health during crises

In the realm of social sciences, the study of mental health during crisis periods is grounded in a set of theories and conceptual models that provide explanatory frameworks for understanding the impact of stressful events on the psychological well-being of individuals and communities. A fundamental theory in this field is the stress and coping theory, developed by Richard Lazarus and Susan Folkman (Lazarus & Folkman, 1984), which posits that individual reactions to stressful situations are mediated by cognitive appraisals of events and adopted coping strategies. This theory emphasizes the importance of subjective perception of events and individual adaptive capacity, thus providing a basis for understanding the variability in responses to crises.

Urie Bronfenbrenner's ecological systems theory (Bronfenbrenner, 1979) offers a complementary perspective, placing individual experiences within the broader context of interconnected social systems. This approach suggests that mental health during crises is influenced by complex interactions between the individual and various levels of their social environment, allowing for an analysis of risk and protective factors at multiple social levels.

Attachment theory, initiated by John Bowlby (1969), provides a valuable perspective on how interpersonal relationships influence resilience and adaptation during crises. It suggests that attachment styles formed in childhood continue to influence how individuals cope with stress and seek support in their adult relationships, thus contributing to better adaptation and maintenance of mental health in crisis situations.

Cognitive-behavioral theory, originating in the works of Aaron Beck (1967) and Albert Ellis (1995), provides a framework for understanding how thoughts and behaviors influence emotional states during crises. This approach emphasizes the role of cognitive distortions and maladaptive behaviors in maintaining and exacerbating mental health problems, informing interventions that focus on identifying and modifying negative thought patterns and promoting adaptive behaviors.

A more recent perspective is offered by the Post-Traumatic Growth Theory, developed by Richard Tedeschi and Lawrence Calhoun (Tedeschi & Calhoun, 2004). It proposes that, following confrontation with difficult or traumatic life events, some individuals may experience significant positive changes in self-perception, interpersonal relationships, and life philosophy, thus offering an optimistic perspective on the potential for personal growth and resilience in the aftermath of difficult experiences.

The integration of these theories in the study of mental health during crises provides a solid conceptual foundation for understanding the complexity of human responses to extreme stress situations. They underscore the importance of individual, interpersonal, and socio-cultural factors in shaping experience and adaptation to crises, informing the development of public health interventions and policies aimed at promoting resilience and mitigating the negative impact of crises on mental health. For researchers in the social sciences, these theoretical frameworks offer valuable directions for investigating the mechanisms through which crises affect psychological well-being and for identifying effective prevention and intervention strategies..

I.11. Social isolation and loneliness

Social isolation and loneliness represent two interconnected yet distinct social constructs that have gained increasing significance in the field of sociology, particularly medical sociology, in the context of modern society and global demographic transformations. Social isolation refers to the objective absence or significant reduction of an individual's social interactions and connections with other people or the community as a whole. This can be quantified through indicators such as the frequency of social contacts, the extent of social networks, participation in community activities, or the degree of integration into social structures. Loneliness, on the other hand, constitutes a subjective-emotional experience, characterized by the perception of a discrepancy between desirable and actual social relationships of an individual. Social isolation and loneliness do not always present a direct correlation; an individual can be socially isolated without experiencing feelings of loneliness, while another may feel profound loneliness even in the presence of an extensive social network.

Factors contributing to social isolation and loneliness include demographic changes, urbanization, increased workforce mobility, technological advancements, as well as individual factors such as physical and mental health status, socio-economic status, or significant life events. Cultural and social norms also play a role in shaping the perception and management of these experiences.

The impact of social isolation and loneliness on individual health and well-being is considerable. Studies have shown associations between these phenomena and an increased risk of physical health problems, including cardiovascular conditions, immune system dysfunctions, and premature mortality. From a mental health perspective, these conditions are correlated with higher incidences of depression, anxiety, cognitive decline, and suicidal behavior. The effects transcend the individual sphere, affecting social cohesion and economic productivity at a societal level.

Addressing social isolation and loneliness from a social sciences perspective requires a nuanced understanding of the interaction between individual, interpersonal, and structural factors. Attachment theory, social comparison theory, and the life course perspective offer valuable conceptual frameworks for analyzing these phenomena in social and developmental psychology contexts.

Interventions to combat social isolation and loneliness range from individual-level approaches, such as cognitive-behavioral therapies and social skills improvement interventions, to community initiatives and public policies. These include community programs, creating urban environments that promote social connection, improving access to transportation and technology for vulnerable groups, and integrating the prevention of social isolation into public health strategies.

Social isolation and loneliness thus represent significant challenges in contemporary societies, with profound implications for individual health and collective well-being. Addressing these issues requires an interdisciplinary perspective, integrating knowledge from psychology, sociology, anthropology, and political sciences, to develop effective prevention and intervention strategies.

I.12. Anxiety and frustration in times of pandemic

The COVID-19 pandemic has brought to the forefront two psychological phenomena closely linked to human experience in crisis situations: anxiety and frustration. These two emotional states have become ubiquitous in public discourse and individual experiences, reflecting the profound impact of the pandemic on mental health globally. In the context of social sciences, studying anxiety and frustration during the pandemic period offers a unique window for understanding how large-scale events shape individual psychology and social dynamics.

Anxiety, defined as a state of intense worry or fear regarding uncertain future events or situations (APA, 2013), has been significantly amplified by the COVID-19 pandemic. In this context, anxiety has manifested in multiple forms, from fear of infection and concern for one's own health and that of loved ones, to anxiety related to the economic and social consequences of the crisis. The cognitive theory of anxiety suggests that the perception of threat and the evaluation of one's ability to cope with it are key factors in the development and maintenance of anxious states. In the context of the pandemic, prolonged uncertainty, the constant flow of information (often contradictory), and the feeling of lack of control have created fertile ground for the proliferation of anxiety.

Frustration, on the other hand, refers to the negative emotional state that occurs when an individual is prevented from achieving a goal or satisfying a need. During the pandemic period, sources of frustration have been multiple and varied: mobility restrictions, social isolation, disruption of daily routines, loss of professional or educational opportunities, and the inability to plan for the future. The frustration-aggression theory, although contested in its extreme forms, provides a framework for understanding how accumulated frustration can lead to aggressive behaviors or social conflicts, an aspect observed in the increase of social and political tensions in many societies during the pandemic.

The interaction between anxiety and frustration in the pandemic context has created a complex dynamic, with cascading effects on individual and collective well-being. Health-related anxiety has fueled avoidance and isolation behaviors, which in turn have generated frustration due to unmet social and emotional needs. This negative feedback loop has been exacerbated by the prolonged duration of the crisis, leading to what some researchers have termed "pandemic fatigue" - a state of emotional exhaustion and disengagement in response to chronic stress.

Factors influencing levels of anxiety and frustration during the pandemic are diverse and interconnected. At the individual level, personality traits, previous crisis experiences, and personal coping resources have played an important role in modulating emotional responses. Socio-economic factors, such as occupational status, access to medical resources, and social support, have significantly influenced vulnerability to anxiety and frustration. At the societal level, the quality of public communication, the effectiveness of public health measures, and the degree of social cohesion have been determinants in shaping the collective experience of the pandemic.

The impact of pandemic anxiety and frustration has manifested at multiple levels. At the individual level, increases in rates of depression, anxiety disorders, substance abuse, and sleep problems have been observed. Interpersonal relationships have been strained by isolation, conflicts related to adherence to safety measures, and divergences in risk perception. At the community level, accumulated frustration has fueled protest movements and resistance to public health measures, while anxiety has contributed to stigmatizing and discriminatory behaviors.

Addressing anxiety and frustration in the pandemic context requires an interdisciplinary perspective, combining insights from psychology, sociology, anthropology, and political science. Individual-level interventions, such as mindfulness techniques, cognitive-behavioral therapy, and stress management strategies, have proven effective in alleviating anxiety symptoms and managing frustration. At the community level, social support initiatives, mental health education programs, and efforts to build collective resilience have played a crucial role.

The pandemic has also highlighted the importance of public policies in managing mental health on a large scale. Integrating mental health considerations into crisis response planning, improving access to mental health services, and developing effective communication strategies for reducing anxiety and managing public expectations have become priorities for many governments.

The study of anxiety and frustration during the pandemic period offers a perspective through which we can examine human resilience in the face of adversity, social dynamics during crises, and the role of institutions in shaping collective emotional responses. As societies navigate the post-pandemic transition, the lessons learned from this period will be crucial for developing more effective strategies for managing mental health in the face of future global crises. Future research in the social sciences should focus on understanding the long-term effects of pandemic anxiety and frustration, identifying factors that promote resilience in the face of chronic stress, and developing scalable interventions for improving psychological well-being in contexts of prolonged uncertainty.

I.13. Vulnerable groups and risk factors

The COVID-19 pandemic has brought to the forefront the importance of understanding and addressing social vulnerabilities in health crisis situations. The concepts of vulnerable groups and risk factors provide an essential framework for analyzing the differentiated impact of the pandemic on various segments of society and for developing effective policies and interventions.

Vulnerable groups are defined as those segments of the population that, due to specific social, economic, demographic, or geographic characteristics, are exposed to a higher risk of being negatively affected by a crisis or adverse event (Miftode, 2010). In the pandemic context, vulnerability manifests both in terms of susceptibility to infection and reduced capacity to cope with the social and economic consequences of the crisis.

The main vulnerable groups identified during the COVID-19 pandemic include:

• The elderly - They present an increased risk of severe complications and death in case of infection, but are also vulnerable to social isolation and mental health problems as a result of distancing measures.

• People with pre-existing medical conditions - Including cardiovascular diseases, diabetes, chronic respiratory conditions, which are associated with an increased risk of complications in case of COVID-19 infection.

• Ethnic and racial minorities - In many countries, these groups have been disproportionately affected by the pandemic, reflecting pre-existing structural inequalities in access to healthcare and socio-economic conditions.

• Low-income individuals - They are more likely to work in jobs that do not allow telework, have limited access to healthcare, and often live in conditions that facilitate virus transmission.

• Homeless people - Who face difficulties in complying with hygiene and social distancing measures and have limited access to medical services.

• Essential workers - Including medical personnel, food retail workers, and transportation workers, who are exposed to an increased risk of infection due to the nature of their work.

• Children from disadvantaged families - Affected by school closures and the transition to online education, which has exacerbated educational inequalities.

• People with disabilities - Who may face additional barriers in accessing public health information and medical services.

• Migrants and refugees - Often living in precarious conditions and with limited access to health services (Sandu, 2020).

Risk factors contributing to the vulnerability of these groups in a pandemic context are multiple and interconnected:

• Socio-economic factors - Poverty, lack of health insurance, precarious housing conditions, and limited access to information and education resources.

• Occupational factors - Type of work, inability to work from home, and increased exposure to the public.

• Health factors - Presence of chronic diseases, limited access to preventive and curative medical services.

• Demographic factors - Age, gender, and family structure.

• Geographic factors - Living in dense urban areas or isolated rural communities with limited access to medical services.

• Cultural and linguistic factors - Barriers in accessing and understanding public health information.

• Psychological factors - Chronic stress, social isolation, and pre-existing mental health problems.

The impact of the pandemic on vulnerable groups has manifested in multiple dimensions: in the physical realm - higher rates of infection, severe complications, and mortality among certain groups; in the mental health realm - increased incidence of depression, anxiety, and other mental health issues as a result of isolation and economic stress; in the economic realm - job losses, reduced incomes, and increased financial insecurity; in the educational realm - disruption of education and widening educational gaps, especially for children from disadvantaged backgrounds; in the social realm - exacerbation of social isolation, especially for the elderly and people with disabilities.

Addressing vulnerabilities in a pandemic context requires an intersectional perspective that recognizes how different forms of disadvantage intersect and amplify each other. This understanding is crucial for developing effective policies and interventions that address not only the symptoms but also the root causes of vulnerability.

Public policy responses during the pandemic have included:

- ✓ Social protection measures: Expansion of social assistance programs and introduction of financial support schemes for affected groups.
- ✓ Targeted communication strategies: Development of culturally and linguistically adapted information materials for diverse groups.
- ✓ Public health interventions: Priority testing and vaccination campaigns for high-risk groups.
- ✓ Housing policies: Measures to prevent evictions and ensure safe shelters for homeless individuals.
- ✓ Educational support: Programs to support distance learning and reduce the digital divide.
- ✓ Mental health initiatives: Expansion of psychological support services and promotion of mental health.

For researchers in the social sciences, the study of vulnerable groups and risk factors in a pandemic context offers significant opportunities to examine and reduce structural inequalities in society.

The analysis of vulnerable groups and risk factors in a pandemic context underscores the importance of a holistic and equitable approach in managing public health crises. This requires close collaboration between different disciplines of social sciences, such as sociology, anthropology, psychology, and political science, as well as an integration of these perspectives with medical and public health fields. Through a deep understanding of vulnerabilities and risk factors, societies can develop more effective and equitable strategies to address current and future challenges in public health and social well-being.

I.14. Specialized literature dedicated to the Covid-19 pandemic

The specialized literature in the field of socio-human sciences dedicated to the effects of the Covid-19 pandemic is particularly rich and current. At a first check in Web of Science, on June 21, 2021, a number of 64,847 papers were registered for the topic of the Covid-19 pandemic ("Covid pandemic"). Of these, 4,066 papers are indexed for the keywords "Covid pandemic and anxiety", which shows a particularly broad concern for studying the psychological effects of the pandemic from the perspective of the anxiety state it generates. A more refined search for the keywords "Covid pandemic and social anxiety" yielded a result of 1,566 papers on this topic. Compared to these results, only 102 articles were found for the keywords "Covid pandemic and frustration", which shows a lesser interest in approaching the pandemic from the perspective of frustrations generated among the population. A number of 18 results were identified for the keywords "Covid pandemic and anguish", while 399 results were found for the keywords "Covid pandemic and panic".

Conducting a general meta-analysis on the topic of stress, anxiety, and depression among the population during the Covid-19 pandemic, Nader Salari and colleagues (Salari et al., 2020) show that this epidemic has generated a significant number of psychological disorders, which were added to the actual concern about the physical health state of the population. The mentioned study shows that the spread of the virus has a significant impact on the population from various communities and, therefore, during the pandemic, psychological measures must be taken to improve the mental health of the population, especially vulnerable groups. The mentioned research appeared on July 6, 2020, and analyzed papers published in journals indexed in various databases until May 2020. Data on the prevalence of stress resulting from the pandemic were collected by analyzing five studies, on a total sample of 9,074 people, resulting in an incidence of 29.6% of stress among the studied population. The prevalence of anxiety was analyzed according to 17 studies conducted during the mentioned period, on a sample of 63,439 people, with the level of anxiety affecting 31.9% of the investigated population. The prevalence of depression was analyzed based on 14 studies, conducted on a total sample of 44,531 people, being rated at a level of 33.7% of these.

Comparing these results with the incidence of anxiety in the United States in 2013, according to DSM-5, previously mentioned to be 13.3%, we can notice a worrying increase in this disorder, due to the emergence of the pandemic. At the time of the mentioned study, it was known that Covid-19 infection generates a symptomatology that includes fever, chills, cough, sore throat, muscle pain, nausea, and vomiting. Infected persons manifested symptoms of varying severity, from simple cold symptoms - later medically documenting situations of infected but asymptomatic persons - to severe cases, manifesting respiratory failure or acute respiratory syndrome, which can culminate in the patient's death. Salari and his collaborators' article focuses on the psychological effects of the pandemic - not of the actual Covid-19 infection - effects highlighted at the individual, community, national, or international level during the period when most states were in lockdown.

At the individual level, the authors of the cited study, based on previous literature dedicated to pandemics (Hall et al., 2008), considered as predictable individual behaviors in which subjects manifest states of fear generated by the possibility of their own death or that of close persons, by the feeling of helplessness and the obligation to manifest stereotypical social behavior (Salari et al., 2020). The harmful effect of the pandemic at the psychological level, the authors of the cited study draw our attention, can generate a significant psychological crisis, which can be considered a real threat to public mental health (Xiang et al., 2020).

The effect of the psychological crisis is considered to be more pronounced in the case of patients manifesting the incipient stages of mental disorders, the major health crisis determined by the Covid-19 pandemic potentially leading to psychological changes including at a pathological level, both for healthcare personnel and for citizens. The most probable pathologies or disorders are determined by fear, anxiety, depression, or insecurity (Zhang et al., 2020).

Research consulted by Salari and colleagues demonstrates that people in isolation and quarantine manifest significant levels of anxiety, anger, confusion, and stress (Brooks et al., 2020). Also, studies conducted in the early stages of the spread of the Covid-19 virus in Asia show that fear regarding the spread of the virus, especially in the context of lack of information about its nature (infection rate, morbidity, mortality), can lead to mental disorders, including severe ones (Shigemura et al., 2019). The predisposition for mental disorders and even mental illnesses is accentuated in the case of certain social categories, which include patients infected with Covid-19 and their families, healthcare workers, children, and patients with other mental disorders (Bao et al., 2020).

Another study on the prevalence of anxiety and depression during the Covid-19 pandemic was conducted among students from healthcare faculties in Jordan (Basheti et al., 2021). The study highlights a series of particularities regarding the prevalence of anxiety and depression when referring to healthcare personnel involved in one form or another in the direct care of patients infected with Covid-19, personnel who, for this reason, present a high degree of risk of contracting the virus. The cited study shows that there is, indeed, a high level of anxiety among the surveyed students. Among the persons psychologically tested through an online survey, based on the Hospital Anxiety and Depression Scale (HADS), 40% of participants recorded normal scores for anxiety and depression, 22.4% obtained a borderline normal score, while 33.8% of the surveyed students had a score considered abnormal regarding anxiety, and 26.2% of respondents had an abnormal score regarding depression. Other anxiogenic factors were also taken into account, such as smoking, low family income, and the use of specific medication, which showed a statistically significant correlation with anxiety. After excluding these additional anxiogenic factors, the percentage of persons with high levels of anxiety remained significantly increased compared to the normal from periods before the pandemic.

The specialized literature analyzes the impact of the Covid-19 pandemic on the incidence of migraines and other neurological disorders (Suzuki et al., 2021). Suzuki and colleagues show that the

Covid-19 pandemic has generated a series of neurological disorders, including migraines, sleep disorders, anxiety, and depression. These disorders were recorded especially during the first wave of the pandemic, with subsequent waves not bringing significant variations regarding the occurrence of these types of disorders. Also, during the first pandemic wave, a significant increase in the consumption of neuroleptics was recorded, following the increase in stress levels, in parallel with the identification of comorbidities associated with Covid-19. Studies cited by Suzuki and colleagues (Suzuki et al., 2021) also show that there was a significant impact of changing social conditions in various countries (social distancing, lockdown, diminished social mobility and freedom of travel) on people who were not actually infected with Covid-19 (Ozamiz-Etxebarria et al., 2020). An increase in the negative impact of the pandemic on hospitalized patients with migraines and acute headaches was also noted (Kristoffersen et al., 2020). Other works consulted by the same team of researchers highlight the concerns of American psychiatrists regarding the interruption of treatment for patients with mental disorders, including those with migraines, interruption caused by the postponement of non-emergency therapies, which were imposed by many states to limit Covid-19 infection (Rizzoli & Grazzi, 2020).

We insisted on presenting these results to demonstrate the acute nature of some mental disorders that occurred during the Covid-19 pandemic and which severely affected the quality of life of psychiatric or neurological patients, but also of people who do not usually suffer from mental disorders, regardless of whether they were diagnosed with Covid-19 or not.

Other research investigates the predictive role of intolerance to uncertainty - regarding family life, marital status, children, health status, chronic diseases, elderly in care, relatives working in healthcare, the existence of relatives or close persons diagnosed with Covid-19 infection, etc., all these categories being perceived to be at risk of infection - on the occurrence of depression and anxiety in people physically or socially affected by the pandemic (Korkmaz & Güloğlu, 2021). The results of the mentioned research showed that the meaning of life and intolerance to uncertainty were significant predictors of depression and anxiety. Chronic disease is a significant predictor of anxiety, and hand washing frequency is a significant predictor of depression. It was concluded that the most important variables influencing both depression and anxiety were intolerance to uncertainty and the meaning of life.

Cap. II. Anxiety and frustration due to the pandemic - qualitative research

The research aimed to highlight the phenomena of anxiety and anguish due to restrictions imposed during the pandemic.

II.1. Research objectives

The research objectives are represented by:

- Understanding the changes that Romanian families are experiencing due to the pandemic;
- Identifying the elements of social construction of the idea of pandemic and infodemic, in the context of the public health crisis;
- Highlighting and analyzing potential manifestations and risks created by anxiety and frustration - emerging during the pandemic period;

- Identifying the specifics of social perception regarding the pandemic among the population in the North-East Region of Romania.

II.2. Research hypotheses

For our research, the hypotheses (presuppositions) are:

- **Hypothesis 1**: The Coronavirus (Covid-19) pandemic has negatively influenced the mental health state of the population, inducing states of anguish and anxiety among a significant portion of the population.
- **Hypothesis 2:** The lockdown measures associated with the Covid-19 pandemic will influence the prosocial behaviors of individuals, depending on the severity of the anguish experienced by them during the implementation of these measures.
- **Hypothesis 3:** The transformations that society has undergone at the cultural, economic, and communicational levels can lead to an intensification of the medicalization of social life.

II.3. Sample and actual conduct of the research

The research took place between April-June 2020, at national level (in Romania), on a sample of 103 people, predominantly in the N.E. region of Romania (67) as follows: Suceava (42), Botosani

(15), Iasi (10), but also from other counties: Cluj (1), Bucharest (2). People from the Republic of Moldova (12) were also interviewed, as well as Romanian citizens domiciled in other countries such as: Austria (1), Spain (1), Italy (1), Belgium (1), Germany (1), United Kingdom (1). There were also people who did not declare their region/country of residence: unspecified (15).

The interviewed persons were female (62), male (31), and 7 people did not specify their gender.

The age of the interviewed persons ranges between 18-24 years (47), 25-30 years (26), 35-45 years (14), 45-60 years (9), 60-90 years (3), unspecified (4).

As for the background, the interviewed persons belong to rural areas (42), urban areas (25), unspecified (36).

Regarding the level of education, research participants declared as formal education higher studies (63) and secondary studies (31), unspecified (9).

The occupational profiles of the persons included in the sample were as follows: salesperson (7), medical staff (6), student (35), pupil (9), teacher (5), economist (3), clerk (1), civil servant (10), commerce worker (3), unemployed (4), housewife (6), retired (7), unspecified (7).

The sample was one of opportunity, the sample selection being made based on the snowball method, and the analysis of the collected data took into account the need for theoretical saturation of the proposed model (no new discursive categories were identified in the following interviews). In fact, the saturation of the model was achieved in general lines after analyzing the first 20 interviews, but the analysis continued, identifying significant subcategories which, although they did not bring new discursive categories, better configured the existing categories.

The research was conducted based on unstructured interviews, applied online or by phone (Sandu, 2021). For the most part, the interviews were conducted through video conferencing applications and were transcribed. A limited number of interviews were conducted through Messenger, WhatsApp programs - where both questions and answers took place in writing, the answers being given by the interviewed persons immediately after receiving the question - thus ensuring real-time communication. The interviews mainly aimed to highlight how the families of students, as well as those of their friends and acquaintances, related to the situation created by the pandemic.

We mention that during the period when the research was conducted, both Romania and the other countries of origin of the respondents were in a lockdown period, characterized by the closure of non-essential economic activities, limiting the mobility of persons through the obligation of a self-declaration regarding the purpose, duration and route of travel, the complete prohibition of travel between certain time intervals or even the complete quarantine of persons suspected of infection with SARS-COV-2 or of entire localities where the infection rate was increased compared to the national average.

II.4. The methodological dimension of the research

Grounded Theory (GT) represents a distinct qualitative research methodology that has gained significant importance in the field of social sciences (Sandu, 2018). This methodological approach is characterized by its exploratory nature and the ability to generate explanatory theoretical constructs based directly on empirical data collected from the field, rather than on pre-existing hypotheses derived from literature. In contrast to traditional research paradigms that aim to verify predefined theories or hypotheses, the primary objective of GT is to generate new theoretical frameworks regarding the studied social phenomena through a predominantly inductive process.

From a social-constructionist epistemological perspective, GT emphasizes the multiple and contextual nature of social reality, highlighting the active role of the researcher in co-constructing knowledge with study participants. This approach recognizes that the results of the investigation are inextricably linked to the specific context of the research, thus inverting the logic of classical scientific inquiry by abandoning the primary reference to gaps identified in the literature and adopting a directly exploratory attitude towards empirical data.

The methodological process of GT involves a series of interconnected and iterative steps. Theoretical sampling and data collection are carried out simultaneously, without predetermining the sample size. This process continues until theoretical saturation is reached, at which point new data no longer generate novel categories or conceptual relationships. Open or initial coding represents the first stage of interpretation, conducted through meticulous analysis of data transcripts, identifying primary codes and formulating memos - theoretical reflections of the researcher on the analyzed data.

Axial coding involves grouping primary codes into more comprehensive semantic categories, exploring relationships between them to construct a preliminary analytical model. Selective coding aims to establish the central category and refine inter-categorical relationships, with the goal of elevating the model to a higher degree of generality, transcending the specific context of the research. The constant comparison principle, fundamental in GT, involves continuous comparative analysis of data, codes, and categories, both among themselves and in relation to existing theories in the literature.

Evaluation of the resulting theoretical model is conducted through the lens of its credibility, rather than statistical validity, this plausibility being strengthened through triangulation of interpretations, methodologies, and data sources. In conclusion, GT generates hypotheses instead of definitive conclusions, these key statements of the theoretical model potentially constituting premises for subsequent quantitative investigations.

The applicability of GT in various domains of social sciences is illustrated through concrete examples, such as the study of professional experience of diabetologists and the social construction of chronic illness. In such a study, through focus groups with specialists in diabetology, the researcher can explore how clinical experience shapes medical perceptions and practices, as well as how chronic illness is conceptualized and managed in a social context.

In essence, Grounded Theory provides a flexible yet rigorous methodological framework for exploring and theorizing complex social phenomena, allowing us to generate innovative explanatory models firmly anchored in the studied empirical reality. This approach was particularly utilized due to the exploratory nature of the research in investigating little-explored domains or in critically re-examining existing concepts and theories in social sciences.

II.5. Analysis of results using Grounded Theory method

For data interpretation, the qualitative analysis methodology called *Grounded Theory* (G.T.) was utilized (Corbin & Strauss, 2008; Creswell, 2007; Goulding, 1999). The method consists of a systematic process of generating conceptual categories, aiming to achieve an increasingly higher level of generality that explains the researched theme. The approach is inductive, through successive work stages, starting from the information provided by the interviewed subjects. The research generally has an exploratory character, being used when investigating a novel psycho-social phenomenon, about which there is insufficient data in the specialized literature or for which existing theories in the literature are no longer applicable due to changes in the socio-cultural contexts in which the social phenomenon occurs. This approach is frequently used in social psychology, as well as in sociology, cultural studies, public health, etc.

Due to the exploratory nature of the method, it aims to create a new theoretical corpus rather than validating a set of prior hypotheses (Corbin & Strauss, 2008; Sandu, 2010). Hypotheses can exist in the form of presuppositions, derived either from literature or from an initial empirical analysis of the studied social phenomenon, but the research does not have an actual confirmatory value, this type of research being limited to highlighting possible causal links, without being able to effectively confirm them and without being able to precisely specify the causal dynamics of the social phenomenon.

The results thus obtained will be synthesized in the form of a model, whose constituent elements, formulated as possible causal relationships, can constitute working hypotheses for future research. These would aim to clarify the resulting model, as well as the extent of its validity.

Data coding was carried out in two successive phases: initial coding and, respectively, selective - focused (Adam, 2009) - coding, which we called, in accordance with, axial coding. The purpose of these successive inductive stages is to identify significant themes or discursive categories, followed by the construction of an explanatory theoretical model of social phenomena accompanying anxiety and frustration, which emerged as an effect of the pandemic, but also of the measures to prevent Covid-19 infection. The classification of obtained "codes" or categories and the reunification of initial categories that are semantically adjacent was pursued. In the first stage, open coding was used, followed, within the analysis process, by axial coding (Corbin & Strauss, 2008), where, from the thematic axes, a series of theoretical constructs with an explanatory role resulted in the elaboration of an instrumental model for understanding the dimensions perceived by the population of social phenomena related to the pandemic, as well as possible pathologies generated by anxiety and frustration.

Cap. III. Anxiety and distress during the pandemic. Research results

The primary data analysis corresponds to the *open coding stage*, a stage at which each interview was analyzed, identifying key words and phrases and, subsequently, significant semantic categories. As a result of the axial coding process, 16 categories emerged, as follows:

Category	Subcategories	No. of in-vivo codes
Information regarding the Covid-19 virus/pandemic	Online	12
	Traditional mass-media	17
	From other people	6
	From infected people	3
	Sufficiently informed	5
	Insufficiently informed	5

Personal experience of infection with Covid-19 virus	Personal	1
	Close relatives	3
	Suspicions of infection	5
Experience of communicating with people infected with Covid-19 virus / quarantined and perception of them	People infected with Covid-19	4
	Quarantined people (contact or local quarantine)	6
	Quarantined people with comorbidities	1
Subjective experience of quarantine measures, social distancing and lockdown	Quarantine and lockdown (due to general measures in force)	23
	Personalized quarantine after returning from abroad	2
	Social distancing	18
	Lack of access to public places and events	10
	Limitation of access to religious services	5
	Limitation of access to medical/health services	4
	Relationships with close persons and sociability	19
	Decrease in quality of life	16
	Obligation of self-declaration*	6
	Change in lifestyle	21
	Loss of job	4
	Financial situation	8
	Limitation of civil rights	4

<table>
<tr><td rowspan="7">Relation to restrictive measures imposed by authorities during the pandemic</td><td colspan="2">Acceptability</td><td>26</td></tr>
<tr><td colspan="2">Unacceptability</td><td>7</td></tr>
<tr><td colspan="2">Compliance</td><td>32</td></tr>
<tr><td colspan="2">Non-compliance</td><td>5</td></tr>
<tr><td colspan="2">Efficiency</td><td>15</td></tr>
<tr><td colspan="2">Inefficiency</td><td>12</td></tr>
<tr><td colspan="2">Ambivalence</td><td>9</td></tr>
<tr><td rowspan="4">Perception regarding the existence of necessary resources to overcome the pandemic</td><td rowspan="2">At individual level</td><td>Positive</td><td>4</td></tr>
<tr><td>Negative</td><td>9</td></tr>
<tr><td rowspan="2">At community/ societal level</td><td>Positive</td><td>2</td></tr>
<tr><td>Negative</td><td>11</td></tr>
<tr><td rowspan="15">Relation to the severity of Covid-19 virus: anguish and anxiety</td><td colspan="2">Anguish / Anxiety</td><td>29</td></tr>
<tr><td colspan="2">Frustration</td><td>17</td></tr>
<tr><td colspan="2">Stress</td><td>12</td></tr>
<tr><td colspan="2">Hopelessness</td><td>2</td></tr>
<tr><td colspan="2">Revolt</td><td>2</td></tr>
<tr><td colspan="2">Instability</td><td>6</td></tr>
<tr><td colspan="2">Depression</td><td>2</td></tr>
<tr><td colspan="2">Disappointment</td><td>2</td></tr>
<tr><td colspan="2">Insecurity</td><td>2</td></tr>
<tr><td colspan="2">Fluctuation of emotional state</td><td>2</td></tr>
<tr><td colspan="2">Sources of anguish</td><td>15</td></tr>
<tr><td colspan="2">Sources of frustration</td><td>13</td></tr>
<tr><td colspan="2">Moment of awareness</td><td>23</td></tr>
<tr><td colspan="2">Correctness of assessment vs. exaggeration of pandemic severity</td><td>3</td></tr>
</table>

	Did not experience states of anguish or anxiety		10
	Dangerousness of the virus	high	16
		low	4
	Fight against the virus/pandemic		2
Impact of news regarding the pandemic	Positive		1
	Negative		20
	No impact		1
Perceived effects of the pandemic	Positive		20
	Negative		26
Credibility of information sources and infodemic	Credible		2
	Not credible		14
Perception regarding the post-pandemic period	Return to normality		6
	Post-pandemic society		21
The post-pandemic immediateness	Recovery of intimacy		1
	Recovery of sociability		2
Transfer of daily activities to online	Changes in lifestyle		6
	Virtualization of social interactions - as a facilitator of communication		9
	Virtualization of social space - form of alienation and social isolation		3
	Lack of necessary resources		2
	Chaotic activity		2

<table>
<tr><td rowspan="5">Protection measures proposed by the interviewed persons</td><td colspan="2">Disinfectant substances</td><td>7</td></tr>
<tr><td colspan="2">Mask and gloves</td><td>14</td></tr>
<tr><td colspan="2">Preventive testing</td><td>1</td></tr>
<tr><td colspan="2">Maintaining calm and lucidity</td><td>8</td></tr>
<tr><td colspan="2">Social distancing</td><td>9</td></tr>
<tr><td rowspan="5">Relation to the pandemic situation proposed by the interviewed persons</td><td colspan="2">Deepening religious/ spiritual practices</td><td>2</td></tr>
<tr><td colspan="2">Writing a journal about experiences during the pandemic</td><td>1</td></tr>
<tr><td colspan="2">Presence of companion animals</td><td>3</td></tr>
<tr><td colspan="2">Recreational activities reading, watching movies, listening to music</td><td>10</td></tr>
<tr><td colspan="2">Gymnastics, indoor physical activities</td><td>2</td></tr>
<tr><td rowspan="6">Conspiracy theories regarding the pandemic and Coronavirus</td><td rowspan="2">Biological weapon / synthetic origin of the virus</td><td>Yes</td><td>3</td></tr>
<tr><td>No</td><td>1</td></tr>
<tr><td colspan="2">Pandemic as a source of enrichment / pharma industry</td><td>1</td></tr>
<tr><td colspan="2">Unconventional war including economic or hybrid</td><td>2</td></tr>
<tr><td colspan="2">A New World Order</td><td>1</td></tr>
<tr><td colspan="2">Non-existence of the virus</td><td>1</td></tr>
<tr><td rowspan="2">Perception of the pandemic</td><td colspan="2">Personification of the virus / animistic attitude</td><td>1</td></tr>
<tr><td colspan="2">Teleological perspective</td><td>5</td></tr>
</table>

*The document, in Romania, was called „***Declaration on one's own responsibility***”. We have used, in our text, the juridical term „affidavit”, respectively the more common term „self-declaration”, more frecvently used from sociological point of view.

III.1. Information on the Covid-19 virus / pandemic: origins, cause, manifestation, treatment

The interviewed persons have an ambivalent opinion regarding the pandemic, with the majority considering themselves ***sufficiently informed*** (S.D.B.) from online sources (A.A.), (D.A.B.), (G.F.C.), as well as from traditional mass media (L.B.), (G.F.C.), (B.S.A.). Some of them indicate that they consider themselves *sufficiently* informed about the symptoms that Covid-19 infection can present: *fever, dry cough* (A.A.), while other individuals show that they have knowledge only about the severity of the disease, but not about its manifestations: they only know that it affects the body very strongly (D.A.B.).

For some respondents, a credible source of information regarding the manifestations and symptoms of the disease is ***communication with infected persons***, especially those who have gone through the illness and managed to overcome it. In this case, the information obtained can constitute a source of ***optimism and confidence*** that the disease can be overcome. (I.E.). The same is not true when the close person infected with Covid-19 has lost their life. In such cases, the interviewed subjects deeply realize the ***risks*** that SARS-COV-2 infection can bring, both for themselves and for those close to them, especially if it concerns elderly persons or those suffering from comorbidities (S.P.).

To avoid ***misinformation*** that appears due to the abundance of information sources, many of them contradictory, some individuals have decided to ***select their information sources***, giving credibility especially to medical and scientific sources, as well as personal accounts of patients who have recently gone through the disease: *The sources of information were varied, internet, mass media, magazines, and newspapers. This avalanche of information initially scared me, because I didn't know what to believe, as many of them contradicted each other. I started to follow the opinion of doctors, researchers, and people who have been infected by this virus* (I.E.).

III.2. Personally experiencing Covid-19 infection

A significant experience mentioned by the interviewed subjects was that of ***their own infection with the Covid-19 virus*** and, respectively, situations where close persons were infected with this virus. When there were individuals among those close to them who lost their lives due to infection with the virus, ***the described experience*** was one of ***anguish*** for their own health state and, especially, for that of their loved ones: *When I found out that one of our family acquaintances was contaminated with this virus, and after a few days of hospitalization died...*

They were elderly, it's true, 76 years old and suffering from several illnesses. But that was the moment when I became quite worried for my family as well (S.P.). Another person, who had close relatives infected with the SARS-COV-2 virus, considers these individuals to be the most credible source of information regarding the virus manifestations and disease symptoms, but also a source of optimism and confidence when these close persons successfully overcome the illness: *My aunt is a nurse at a hospital in Milan, a heavily affected area. She had the misfortune of confronting SARS-COV-2, so I managed to find out more details about the symptoms of this viral infection, from the perspective of an infected person. It was a very difficult period, she had a fever of 39 degrees Celsius, chills, fatigue, muscle pain, headache. Now she has resumed her activity with more confidence and optimism* (I.E.).

III.3. Experience of communicating with people infected with Covid-19 virus and perception upon them

A series of ***communication experiences with persons infected*** with the Covid-19 virus were highlighted (L.B.), with manifestations of different intensity and severity, from individuals who went through this experience easily and recovered, to those who suffered physically and psychologically, for whom the infection was a ***traumatic experience***. The interviewed subjects showed that among their more or less close acquaintances, there were also people who *lost the battle with the virus* (A.A.).

Towards infected persons, feelings of ***empathy*** and even ***joy*** are manifested, when they prove to be ***cured*** (A.A.). Responses such as *Yes, I have acquaintances who had such persons in their family and were forced to stay in quarantine, but this has not changed in any way how I behave with them. Everything remained exactly as before, the virus cannot change who you are* (L.B) are worth noting. Such statements represent true pleas against discrimination of infected persons - ***discrimination*** that could arise, on one hand, due to ***social fear*** of infection and infected persons but, on the other hand, can also be induced by ***the severity of quarantine measures***, both for individuals (quarantined individually as mere contacts of these) and for some communities (at which level the virus spread rate is higher than the national average).

Direct contact with an infected person, especially when that person's case appeared in the media, becomes a source of anguish and even ***despair***, the interviewed subject being concerned about their ***own health condition***, but also about the possibility of themselves being a ***vector of virus transmission***: *The moment I realized that this virus had reached the locality where I live, I got quite scared, because, first of all, I had contact with a person who had contact with the first Covid case in the locality. Then, numerous news appeared where it was presented that this person infected another 1000 people, which has now proven false. I started to* *worry for my loved ones, but also for myself, I started to refuse to follow the news anymore, because they induced panic in me and, even at present, I avoid them. I had periods when I felt like isolating myself, I cried, I felt helpless and I got very scared, but at present I am better and with more hope. [...] Social distancing affected me, first of all, in that two-week period when my family and I stayed isolated, because we thought we had contact with that person I mentioned earlier* (B.A.G.).

III.4. The subjective experience of quarantine, social distancing and lockdown measures

The ***subjective experience*** of quarantine depends on how individuals perceive the risks that the disease for which quarantine was imposed can bring to their own life and that of their loved ones, and only then the impacts it brings to their own freedoms, lifestyle, and agency capacity. People who feel more vulnerable - due to age or ***comorbidities*** - may be more inclined to accept stricter quarantine measures or even adopt for themselves and their loved ones a quarantine lifestyle that, out of precaution, exceeds the minimum measures imposed by authorities: *I easily accepted the idea of self-isolation, because I would have chosen it even if it hadn't been imposed, as it seems to me a safe method to protect my health, because the risks are much higher in the case of the condition I have, namely I am a type I insulin-dependent diabetic, and this disease has brought with it a multitude of fears and insecurities* (G.G.).

The modification of lifestyle, whether in a sense considered agreeable or disagreeable, represents the representative subjective experience of the interviewed persons when they refer to quarantine measures, social distancing, and lockdown: *I had gotten used to a certain lifestyle, and now everything is different* (E.L.). The lockdown period was considered by some people as ***a moment of respite*** in daily activities, which allowed them to dedicate themselves to ***hobbies*** or recreational activities that they would not have allowed themselves in a normal period, such as reading, watching TV or online movies or shows, practicing meditation or prayer, gymnastics, etc. The interviewed person (A.C.) occupied their free time with watching movies, which in our opinion allowed them to detach from alarming news and possible ***sources of frustration*** due to lockdown, in the context where that person considers this period as a period of relaxation before going to work abroad.

Many of the interviewed persons consider that they were affected by the ***imposed restrictions***, one of them declaring that *they hadn't seen their family for two months* (A.A.), but mentions regarding the lack or diminution of relationships with family members or close persons during the quarantine or lockdown period appeared in most interviews. The reason why some of the interviewees declared themselves in agreement with the imposed measures and respected them was the protection of their loved ones and less their own protection.

Opinions were recorded according to which, after relaxing quarantine measures, the number of infected persons will increase greatly. The interviewed persons consider themselves responsible for their own health state, without exaggerating protective measures: *I can't say I exaggerated, but I didn't leave my life to chance either* (D.A.B). The constituent elements of an ordinary life were affected in the case of some respondents, including relationships with friends and, implicitly, their sociability (n.n.), generating *a need to spend more time outdoors* (L.B). In the same direction, some interviewees considered the lockdown period as one in which they had the opportunity ***to dedicate more time to family and loved ones*** (G.N.), with whom they were in quarantine (N.N.1). Spending time with family - which would otherwise have been much diminished - was able to change ***the quality of relationships*** between family members living in the same household, either in the sense of ***strengthening solidarity*** between its members (due to increased communication), or in the sense of ***depreciation of these relationships*** - due to the escalation of latent conflicts, against the background of ***long-term cohabitation obligation***.

There were also confessions of dissatisfaction related to the impossibility of normal conduct of ***special events*** in individuals' lives that would represent unique moments for them. The case brought up is that of graduation banquets and festive courses (S.D.B.), (S.D.), of activities such as enrolling in driving school or traveling abroad (S.D.), as well as other events that had to be postponed - weddings, baptisms - or that had to be conducted with a very small number of participants - funerals. The impossibility of practicing certain ***religious rituals***, including those related to funeral rituals ("mourning the dead"), was also mentioned. ***The restriction of religious freedom***, taken to the total prohibition of public religious services, even during periods of maximum importance holidays for believers of all religions, was considered a serious cause for concern regarding the respect of ***individual rights***, but also a source of emotional trauma for certain deeply religious persons. *The hardest period during isolation was Easter. We, in the countryside, have our customs, we go to church, to the cemetery, we couldn't get used to the idea that it is forbidden for us* (M.T.). However, there are also voices that welcome this measure, considering it ***beneficial for limiting the infection rate*** (P.I.2).

There were situations where people declare that they experienced quarantine both as a result of their own Covid-19 infection, and preventively, following contact with persons tested positive (S.D.B.) - contact that was not followed by infection. Some interviewed persons showed that they are in ***technical unemployment*** as a result of the ***temporary closure of the activity*** of the company where they had their job, this situation constituting a source of anxiety including regarding the future economic situation (A.B.), (G.F.C.).

The quarantine of close persons represents, in turn, a source of anguish and frustration, especially when those persons represent the main / only source of income for the family, and they do not benefit from technical unemployment or other forms of social assistance: *I am worried that my husband, being in a foreign country very affected by this virus, has to face various obstacles for returning to normality. [...] My husband has been in quarantine for a month and a half already, not being guaranteed any kind of financial support, such as technical unemployment, the situation being just as unclear regarding the resumption of activity* (N.A.).

A source of concern regarding the worsening of health during the pandemic and as an indirect effect of the pandemic is ***the issue of mental health***, which is considered to be deteriorated by the ***lack of direct communication*** with others, the ***monotony of activities*** and ***mental fatigue*** (G.N.) *Home isolation made everything difficult and depressing* (L.A.E.). Among the mentioned effects were also those related to the ***decrease in the quality of life*** in general and the general state of well-being, including health, with ***sleep dysfunctions*** being noted (for example, A.B.), which once chronic, can lead to the accentuation of already existing health conditions or the appearance of new disorders. Also, the ***subjective quality of life*** was affected by lockdown measures and the ***obligation to stay at home*** - perceived also as a severe restriction of freedom of movement (G.F.C.).

The limitation of freedom of movement, achieved either through quarantining certain areas or through circulation restrictions during certain time intervals, is considered a source of concern and frustration, especially as a series of measures introduced during the state of emergency expressly require that the movement of persons - even in the interval when it is not completely prohibited - be carried out only on the basis of an ***affidavit/ self-declaration***, controllable by authority representatives, specifying the travel itinerary, purpose, and duration. This measure induces a profound ***negative impact***, being associated in the ***collective mindset*** with a ***state of siege*** and the imminence of catastrophes - in this case, a public health catastrophe. *Not having experience with such situations in the past, I had to think, be careful if I had the declaration with me, if I had filled it out, if I was in the corresponding interval, and so on* (V.A.R.). The restriction of freedom of movement itself ***infringes on personal dignity***, lifestyle, and personal liberty, guaranteed by the Constitution and international conventions, which in the collective mindset of a country that has emerged from communism, such as Romania, may suggest the installation of a dictatorship - called by some sources "***White Dictatorship***" or "***Medical Dictatorship***". Especially in the case of minorities who have been subjected to persecutions throughout history, such measures can trigger ***negative emotional stimuli*** related to ***personal security***, especially in the context where images of law enforcement ensuring compliance with lockdown measures were accessible at least online and quite viewed by the public. The impact of these images was amplified by the - desired or not - deficient communication from the authorities, which through "Military Ordinances" emphasized the martial capacity of the State and less its solidarity with the population. The "***guilt of being infected with Covid-19***" was induced to the population as an idea, even if the purpose of the limiting messages was attributed to the desire to protect the population.

The vulnerability of the population in the face of a ***repressive system*** was highlighted even in the case of a democratic society that accepts and respects human rights, as is the case of the Romanian society where the research was conducted. A social fear, such as that of a pandemic, coupled with inadequate reactions from the authorities, can generate a recoil of freedom, but also an increase in aggressive mentality towards vulnerable populations - such as patients infected with Covid-19. The extension of discrimination towards any person with suspicious symptoms - see the temperature measurement devices present in all public places - can constitute an impetus for ***social segregation***, physical distancing being replaced by ***real social distancing***, not only in terms of maintaining a safety distance, but also in the sense of limiting sociability. All these aspects can have the "perverse" effect of increasing the attitude of ***civic disobedience*** to measures considered abusive or exaggerated in relation to the local dynamics and dimensions of the pandemic. *Some citizens circulate even without self-declarations, whether they have a well-founded reason or not, although the lack of this leads to quite large fines* (P.I.2).

In some situations, a distinction is made between measures designed at the central level, which may be correct, and their application in the territory, which appears to be erroneous, ***unadapted to the concrete situation***, thus arousing the dissatisfaction of citizens, especially in quarantined localities, which have been introduced additional restrictions compared to those faced by the entire population of the country: *As measures to protect the population, initially they were thought out properly, but in the territory they were applied abusively, which led to the revolt of the population* (C.N.E.). Regardless of the level and dimensions at which the pandemic has affected the population, ultimately the ***coping*** capacity of each individual to this ***particular form of stress***, not encountered before, can be defining for overcoming the inconveniences of the period - implicitly anxiety and frustration. It should be noted that the majority of interviewed persons emphasized the ***severity of the crisis***, the discomfort produced, especially in relation to others - to society, to friends, to those close - and less to themselves. Precisely the resistance to anguish and anxiety, by diminishing negative effects and emphasizing positive elements that can be associated with this period, represents such a coping element, which can make those who approach such an attitude overcome these previously mentioned states and any other forms of discomfort more easily, which they mentally positivize, finding possible appreciative elements: *Some were left without money, food. Others gave in psychologically due to pressure and* *stress. It affected us all differently, those with a more open and positive mindset will resist better* (T.S.).

The approach to lockdown can be viewed through the lens of ***social fears***, abundantly present in, practically, all sources of information to which the population has access, or through the lens of a ***moment of respite***, of interruption of daily agitation, of ***return to introspection***, to things that otherwise individuals did not have time to deepen in their relationship with themselves and with those in their immediate vicinity, with whom they were forced to quarantine.

One of the key elements shaping the discourse on the pandemic is that of ***uncertainty*** - both in terms of one's own health and that of loved ones, quality of life, duration of the pandemic and preventive measures, present economic situation, but also in the longer term, etc.: *At the moment, I think uncertainty is the word that describes my state* (A.S.). There were a series of people who showed that during the lockdown period due to the pandemic, they ***lost their job*** - either because they had to give up their job abroad and return to the country, or because the institution or company they worked for temporarily suspended its activity. This unemployment situation, perceived as temporary or long-term, was seen as a source of ***alteration of well-being***, but we consider it necessary to specify that the interviewees make the ***distinction*** between personal well-being, related to ***private life***, and well-being in correlation with the ***workplace***, showing that although they lost their job, they did not feel affected in terms of ***personal state***. This may indicate either an exaggerated optimism related to returning to the labor market as soon as lockdown measures end, or a lack of interest in one's own financial condition, or, very likely, represents a way of showing ***refusal to manifest concern*** for financial condition and stability, which they do not consider defining for their own subjective state of well-being.

Private life is seen as being related to family, friends, and generally to emotional-affective stability, and less to career and ***social expectations*** of the individual - which are perceived as secondary, at the ***periphery of the personality core***. Certainly, this can be connected with various personality factors - which we cannot analyze at this moment because we lack the data - which we can assume exist, at least among young people from certain socio-economic backgrounds, with a distancing from the social model based on evolution on the social ladder and ***job security***, the person's interest transferring to ***emotional security***, experiencing the present moment, and ***immediate satisfaction*** given by daily concrete. The approach to job security, but also to professional evolution, is ***postponed or even neglected*** in favor of ***self-expression***, in the form of being themselves, even if this expression is not necessarily indicated from the perspective of society.

As such, we can conclude that, at least in certain situations, we are not only witnessing a medicalization of social life, but also the emergence of a "***society of personal development***", correlated with the ***dissolution of social solidarity***. ***Interest in***

oneself and those close takes precedence over the interests of society, and jobs are just an alienating element that disturbs the focus on the person. On the other hand, we can notice the existence of a ***culture of precariousness*** and ***focusing on the immediate***, in which individuals refuse long-term planning, to the detriment of living in the immediate.

There were also opinions according to which the pandemic can be considered a ***divine punishment*** for sins accumulated at the level of humanity in general or the community in particular, responsibility being assumed in consonance with a possible ***feeling of guilt***. Divine sanction can, in some situations, be thought of in apocalyptic dimensions, especially since in the collective mindset at least one of the signs of divine wrath is represented by such pandemics. The way the pandemic appeared and its speed of spread globally, the radical and sudden change in lifestyle, the appearance of severe limitations, especially of religious freedom, is sometimes associated with punishment, and people inclined towards such a signification of the pandemic partially experience it as a moment of remembering their own deviations from what they themselves consider - or are socially considered - to be the Divine Will: *Man has always been afraid of a kind of "heavenly punishment" that "will kill us all". Starting from the plague in the Middle Ages to Ebola, and now this virus has appeared which, according to some, will become the end of civilization. Panic and fear appear, which is accompanied by a feeling of helplessness and inability to influence* *what is happening* (A.O.). Divine intervention, for those who see the current pandemic in this way, can have a punitive purpose, as we have presented, but also an educational, corrective one for humanity. *I believe, in fact, that this virus is a sign from God, that we must stop what we are doing, such as all the pollution and, for example, it has been found that many waters have been cleaned as a result of the imposed restrictions, people no longer circulate and, therefore, there is no waste after them. Also, I like to believe that people's consciousness will awaken and we will stop all this chaos, and we will learn to truly appreciate things* (D.I.).

On the other hand, ***belief in divine help*** represents a reason for courage and ***overcoming the uncertainty*** that appears related to the sudden and radical change in lifestyle for an uncertain period of time. *I am not fearful, because I read the holy Bible daily, I pray to God to protect me and my family, and everyone* (P.A.).

Some respondents showed that they feel affected by the pandemic on several levels - personal, social, professional, affective, material, psychological, etc.: *It will affect me on several levels, personally because I don't know if I have escaped the danger of infection, socially because, being a doctor, I have to keep a distance from friends, so as not to predispose them to illness, and professionally, because I am on the threshold of the specialty exam, which I don't know under what conditions it will be held* (C.J.).

III.5. Relating to restrictive measures imposed by authorities during the pandemic

People who declared that they ***accept and even appreciate the protective measures*** requested by the government, state that they also comply with them - they wore masks, gloves, used disinfectant, left the house only when strictly necessary (A.A.), (N.I.). Also, the interviewed persons ***respected social distancing*** as a measure to prevent infection (D.A.B.), (G.F.C.). *Considering that the quarantined areas were the places with the biggest problems, where in some cases they literally exploded, I strongly believe that this measure was wise for all other areas and for all other citizens* (A.M.).

The use of disinfectant and other ***hygiene measures*** are also presented as a form of symbolic distancing - even if unconscious - from others, when the interviewed person emphasizes that, respecting the hygiene measures indicated by the authorities, they disinfect when touching objects that have been touched by other people. (N.N.2). Even if, from a strictly hygienic point of view, this practice reduces the risk of infection, the subjective perception of this gesture reinforces the belief that any person - even if non-present - can be a ***threat***, by simply ***touching objects***. If such a habit is beneficial and salutary during an epidemic crisis in its peak phase, the long-term perpetuation of this habit gives way to a ***perpetuation of social fear towards others***, as a source of risk for one's own health or well-being, which will also strengthen the perception that ***current society is one of risk***, that in fact, not all measures are taken to prevent all risks, which accentuates ***the medicalization of social life***, by accepting the ***inevitability of negative effects in contact with others***. This is all the more true as the same interviewed subject, from whom the above-quoted statement was taken, considers themselves to be as if in prison during the period in which they respond to the interview - the lockdown period in Romania and in the vast majority of countries worldwide: *All the days I stayed in quarantine I felt like a prisoner in my own home, I was afraid to leave the house and, in case I went shopping, I always tried to avoid other people, because I lived in fear that I could catch this virus* (N.N.2).

The ***feeling of imprisonment in one's own home*** is not only related to the restriction of certain rights and freedoms, somewhat understandable in a period of public health crisis, but also to feelings of ***self-blame or blaming others*** for one's own condition, as well as the perception of the ***medicalization of social life as a radicalization of oppression***, in the name of dangers perceived as uncertain. Such a perception can give way to a ***generalized distrust in public health systems***, as vectors of oppression that was once placed exclusively on the political or economic account. A ***complicity*** appears ***between the political, the economic, and the medical***, which in the absence of effective public communication from the authorities, leaves room for ***conspiracy***

theories - some of apocalyptic dimensions. Public entities that assume, in one form or another, opposition to the medicalization of society, or which are perceived to be subject to the same type of oppression during the crisis period, gain special credibility, to the extent that they assume a ***victimhood discourse***. This may involve certain religious elements, vocally manifested by entities that are or legitimize themselves as representatives of religious or political currents in opposition to the exaggerated measures taken by the state.

In most European Union countries, authorities have taken measures to prevent infection, such as lockdown, social distancing, mandatory wearing of masks and gloves, limiting travel outside the home, mandatory self-declaration regarding the purpose, duration, and route of travel, etc. All these measures aimed to reduce the rate of population infection and, in addition to its direct protection, also had the role of avoiding ***overcrowding of hospitals*** with Covid-19 infected patients and, thus, the impossibility of providing medical assistance to all persons who need it.

A contrary opinion was initially embraced by the UK authorities, namely that of achieving ***herd immunity*** by reaching immunity in a large percentage of the population, thus blocking further virus transmission. This opinion was initially supported by the fact that Covid-19, in the form circulating at that time - March to May 2020 - was especially dangerous for people with comorbidities, while other infected individuals could be transmitters but asymptomatic or with symptoms not significantly more severe than those of a cold or flu. The rapid increase in infection rates and the impossibility of systematically protecting people in risk groups led British authorities to abandon this system and adhere to measures applied by most countries worldwide: *Initially, the policy adopted by the government was that of mass immunization, through infection of the entire population. Subsequently, this measure proved to be uncontrollable, the medical system was overloaded and, as a result, measures regarding social distancing were adopted, such as necessary outings to shops, carrying out sports activities, and car travel with a maximum of two people. The activity of all economic agents, local public institutions was suspended, except for agents in the food and pharmaceutical sector. [...] At the moment when there was a massive increase in the number of infected cases at the local level, I was worried about a possible overload of the medical system. That is, if I had been infected or had another health problem, surely the possibilities of addressing a doctor during that period would have been reduced. But now I observe that things have calmed down, and yet we have a considerable number of people who have been cured with the help of medical staff* (B.C.).

The interviewed persons had an ***ambivalent perception*** of the measures taken by authorities, some considering them ***beneficial*** for preventing illnesses and uncontrollable spread of the virus (D.A.B.), while others insisted on the idea that these measures ***were not effective***, that they did not really contribute to reducing the risk of infection (L.B.). The ***disproportionate nature of punitive measures*** imposed in case of non-compliance with quarantine is emphasized, and even ridiculed, compared to other punitive measures in other situations of law violation, but also in relation to the capacity of law enforcement to impose these sanctions: *Thieves and rapists don't end up in prison, do you think those who don't respect isolation will? It's a lie, just to scare those who have recently come to the country* (V.C.).

Others consider that the ***measures*** taken by authorities were ***treated superficially*** (A.A.) by the public. Interviewees consider it a good thing that measures were adopted by the state from the very beginning of the pandemic and that this allowed slowing down the spread of the virus (D.A.B.). There are also criticisms of the measures taken by authorities, considering that *they were not necessarily effective, emphasizing appearances; the situation could have been managed much better* (L.B.). We cannot help but draw attention to this opinion, according to which ***authorities reacted to appearances*** that can be speculated in mass communication - such as wearing masks, social distancing, temperature checks - instead of focusing on ***protecting medical staff***, ensuring necessary and adequate equipment and technology.

There were also opinions according to which ***authorities did not manage*** the social and economic situation during the pandemic ***well enough***, along with technical unemployment measures that appeared in response to the closure of many economic activities. Some criticisms of the state explicitly refer to the lack of medical equipment, which should have existed in hospitals regardless of the occurrence of the current emergency state or not (A.B.). This makes respondents express ***distrust in the state's ability to manage the crisis*** - neither at the health level, nor at the economic and/or social level.

Especially respondents from the Republic of Moldova consider that the authorities in that country are completely incapable of managing the health crisis, which follows years of inefficiencies and dysfunctions of public institutions, and not only those in the health sector (L.C.). The measures proposed by authorities, although criticized as ineffective, are not respected by the population anyway and are applied with delay (in the Republic of Moldova) (L.C.), which allowed the virus to spread to a level where health authorities are no longer able to control this spread through quarantine measures, nor to treat affected persons, with therapeutic needs exceeding the capacity of the health system to cope with the pandemic. Fear of fines and, in general, of the exceptional measures taken during the state of emergency accentuated the state of panic, which was already present among the population (L.C.) in the form of fear of illness, of death - one's own or of loved ones - etc. Through such measures, ***authorities intensified***, on one hand, ***the state of panic and confusion*** among the population, on the other hand, ***they transferred the object of the population's fear*** from the fear of the unknown and fear of death, to the ***fear of authorities*** and the sanctions applied by them, a ***social fear that can be managed*** by complying with legal norms. We base this statement, regarding ***the intentionality of this diversion of public fear*** towards the idea of sanction, precisely on the appearance of ***seemingly irrational and ineffective measures***, such as those related to the need for the affidavit/ the sworn written document when leaving the house, which ***institutes social control*** - and through this a ***public pressure*** - able to partially balance the irrational fear of illness and death, which can only be publicly controlled through preventive measures. Once perceived by the public as effective, this type of measures have the capacity, for a limited period, to calm the state of fear of the population. In this sense, lockdown measures and even quarantine measures, including when they restrict or limit the exercise of fundamental freedoms, are seen by some respondents as beneficial for the health of the population, for preventing the spread of the virus, but also for limiting the anguish of possible infection, precisely by minimizing physical and direct social interactions, with the potential to facilitate virus transmission: *Decisions taken in time, by restricting rights and freedoms, were essential* (A.C.). The interviewed person emphasizes that, due to these measures, Romania's population is less emotionally affected than those of other states, precisely because the number of deaths/illnesses is smaller, largely due to the strictness of the measures and their application since the appearance of the first cases of patients infected with Covid-19: *I believe that all citizens of affected states are equally affected, with low morale. However, our country is maintaining well compared to other states, where the number of deaths is huge* (A.C.).

Authorities thus assume an ***authoritarian but benevolent attitude***, effective in the first period of the pandemic, but ***quickly eroded by public distrust*** and diverted towards the idea of "***white dictatorship***" or dictatorship of public health. It is interesting that an attitude of ***refusal of compliance*** with imposed preventive measures was mentioned even by interviewed persons who declared that they manifested symptoms but refused testing, and also by persons who, being confirmed positive, ***refused hospitalization*** - although at that time it was mandatory -, mentioning ***fear of aggravation of suffering*** in the context of the Romanian health system, considered deficient.

A source of dissatisfaction with the measures taken by authorities to increase the care capacity for Covid-19 patients concerns the transformation of many hospitals into "exclusively Covid" hospitals - which care only for Covid-19 patients - ***leaving without treatment*** or forcing risky and difficult travels for ***patients with other conditions than Covid-19***, endangering their health and even life: *It is annoying for the majority, because not everyone is facing Coronavirus, we don't have so many cases as to "transform" all hospitals, people also have other urgent problems, and traveling to other localities is also risky, depending on the severity of the patient's case* (P.I.2).

Among the interviewed persons, there were some who criticized certain proposals for measures regarding stricter quarantine of elderly persons than the rest of the population, measures that would last even after the relaxation of lockdown measures valid for the rest of the population. These measures are seen as a ***violation of human rights*** and the dignity of these persons[1]. *The wise men of this country are about to send them to camps* [the elderly n.n.]... *God forbid, not extermination camps* (D.S.). Compliance with restrictive measures imposed by authorities is also reinforced by the rather harsh punitive measures that can be applied in case of non-compliance. Fear of sanctions determines some subjects to limit their social contacts outside the home to the strictly necessary: *I don't leave the yard, I talk more with my neighbors, like this over the fence, so that the police don't fine us* (V.C.).

III.6. Perception regarding the existence of the resources necessary to overcome the pandemic

A concern of the interviewed persons is the ***capacity to cope with the pandemic***, from the perspective of the existence or non-existence of medical, human, material, financial resources - both at individual and collective/community or even societal level. Confidence in the existence of resources diminishes the anguish generated by the pandemic,

[1] The measures ultimately remained at public debate level and were never implemented.

while the prospect of insufficient resources can be a source of collective panic.

Situations where people made ***overstocks*** of food and medicines were frequently mentioned, but this panic was somehow stopped when the permanent supply of stores with necessary food products was observed. *My biggest fear was the lack of insulin stock, given the chaos created by the media, at one point there were even news and a commotion around a medicine that did not exist in the pharmacy and there was a much greater concern from this point of view, that I would run out of medicines, which makes my life impossible... medicines make my life possible, without them I could not live and the lack of medicines and food was the first thing that affected me, and the first decision I made was to stock up on insulin for the next three months, to be sure* (G.G. - person suffering from type I insulin-dependent diabetes). The lack of basic necessities and, especially, the fear of complete closure of stores, including food stores, or the impossibility of supplying them were sources of panic declared by several interviewed persons: *At the beginning, when the closure of all stores was announced, we were especially afraid that they would close commercial stores and there was a little panic. In stores then, basic foods, flour, oil, pasta could no longer be found... but we made a small stock and after a week we calmed down and, although we had states of fear, these gradually improved. Now I'm fine* (P.M.).

On the other hand, the lack of protective masks and sanitary equipment - including for medical staff

- was a source of anguish, especially for those who came into direct contact with patients, but also for the entire society. Fears were expressed about the ***insufficiency of medical personnel***, especially when they are subjected to increased risks of infection in the hospital environment, under conditions of insufficient protective equipment and the absence of specific medication or a vaccine[2]. [...] *Doctors are getting sick. Who will treat us? Those who have already been sick are not guaranteed that they will not get sick again* (S.A.). An interviewee even emphasizes, regarding the existence of resources to overcome the pandemic, [...] *For the strictly necessary* [food - n.n] *it is enough, instead the Coronavirus tests [for example] no, and not everyone can afford to do them, from a financial point of view* (P.I.2).

The distrust in the Romanian medical system is attributed by the interviewed persons who chose to respond on this topic to an ***inconsistency of the political factor***, but also to the ***inefficiency of crisis communication*** manifested by the authorities, especially regarding quarantined areas, which seem to be neglected by authorities: *all those* [in orig. in Rom. *others*] *who represent us are incompetent, they don't know how to organize themselves, they don't know how to make wise decisions and ultimately come to the support of Romanian citizens and, unfortunately, with all the regret in the world, I realized that Suceava, for them, represents a*

[2] At the time of the interviews, no vaccine was yet available on the market.

forgotten corner of the world (A.M.). Regarding the previously mentioned response, we cannot certainly separate the effects of frustration vis-à-vis the pandemic and ***the need to find someone responsible*** for the discomfort situation that arose, from the political opinions of the interviewed persons - but the two types of discourse, the political and the personal, converge in the case presented above. The lack of confidence in the medical system is acute also for the interviewed persons living in the Republic of Moldova, due to the insufficiency of medical staff, medical equipment, hospital conditions, etc.: *Almost everything related to the medical system in the country where I am frightens me. The first thing I was thinking about was the fact that in our city there were only two ventilation devices, which means it's insufficient. Also, I was thinking about the unfavorable conditions in which patients are treated, so I also saw a video in which a lady was talking about the lack of equipment at the hospital where those infected with Covid were and were being treated. And the biggest fear was generated by the fact that, out of a number of 900 infected persons at the country level, about 200 cases were among workers in the medical system* (C.I.).

In contrast to the generally negative perception of interviewees from ***Romania*** and the ***Republic of Moldova*** regarding ***the capacity of the medical system*** in these countries to meet the care requirements for persons infected with Covid-19 and, respectively, regarding the ***sanitary safety*** in Romanian hospitals, the interviewed persons of Romanian origin but domiciled in other ***Western European countries*** have confidence that they will be properly cared for, if they were to have the misfortune of being infected with the SARS-COV-2 virus: *I didn't have big fears. The medical system [in this country] is stable, advanced. I had confidence that we would be well treated if we ended up being infected with this virus or if we encountered other problems. But if there had been very many cases, maybe we would have asked some questions. Anyway, we were calm from this point of view* (P.M.).

III.7. Dealing with the severity of Covid-19 virus: anguish and anxiety

In contradiction with our initial presuppositions, according to which the occurrence of states of anguish and anxiety during the pandemic period should be very frequent and we should be able to detect various explicit symptoms of these states - possible ***anxiety disorders*** -, we received quite many responses declaring that research participants ***were not affected*** by the pandemic, but subsequently some of them return and show that they actually lived ***distressing and stressful experiences*** during the pandemic period, but which they do not identify as such and, especially, do not identify in the form of sufferings or disorders, as they do not have obvious external manifestations, but these appear only as changes in mental state or mood, which do not affect self-expression externally (T.E.). For example, the interviewed person T.E. begins by showing that they were not affected by the pandemic, but then specifies that it was very difficult for them, because the lockdown ***changed their way of life*** and they experienced states of anxiety precisely because of these changes.

We consider that responses of this type show that at the level of collective mentality, at least in the studied population, for a person to consider themselves affected by a concrete event, it must drastically change their external state, subjects placing emphasis rather on ***self-expression*** and ***their agent quality***, than on the ***perception of self***, in correlation with the external world, that is, on ***lived experience*** - direct experiencing. As a "synthesis" of the states of anguish and frustration felt by one of the interviewed persons, they declare that: *I somehow felt that my life had disappeared, this truth brought disappointments, frustrations* (I.E.). ***The feeling of loss of life*** - in fact, of its essence -, correlated with the lack of freedom of movement and depreciation of communication, placed the person in ***a situation of non-self***. We understand this state of disappearance of life as an assumption of emblematic elements, which support the ***concrete living of life*** as being life itself, which the subject feels beyond mere biological existence and which they place in ***the cultural and spiritual reality*** in which they are immersed: *I suffered when I could not participate in the funeral of a relative, when I could not hug my loved ones, when that worn mask prevented me from seeing a smile or an expression. I missed the Easter customs and traditions* (I.E.).

A source of stress is represented by the very measures taken by authorities to prevent the spread of the disease, which the subject respects, understanding their necessity, while being aware of the psychological and emotional burden they bring to citizens, both through relating to the awareness of risks, and through the limitations to which citizens are subjected: *I can say that I want to respect these rules from now on too, but I don't know how I will resist psychologically* (B.A.). There were subjects who showed that their ***availability*** and ***emotional state*** changed during the lockdown state, subjects going through periods of intense emotional overexcitement, followed by periods of understanding and acceptance of the situation, fluctuations apparently determined by the information to which the subject has access and the way of interpreting it, but also by the ability to find alternative sources of activity, which require as little movement outside one's own home and limiting physical interactions with other people: *I noticed several changes in my emotional state throughout this period of time. In the first week or, let's say, in the first two weeks, I was very motivated, inspired. In week three, four I was very depressed, bored, a period in which I thought a lot about life, about the meaning of life. Or, in general, we can say that I was thinking too much, I had somewhat gloomier thoughts, accompanied by more depressive behavior and thinking. Subsequently, I adapted, I realized that this pandemic period will not end soon and that things cannot continue like this. I started to inform myself on various topics, which until now did not* *interest me. They might have been interesting for me, but I didn't have enough time and, thus, I didn't get to discover them. So, I decided not to waste time just watching series and movies. A period followed in which I put my thoughts in order and, thus, I became very optimistic, I calmed down, because I started to not follow so much news anymore. The news was always about Coronavirus and, thus, I felt an intention to install fear in people, a state of permanent anxiety* (C.I.).

Regarding the severity of Covid-19 infection and, in general, of the disease triggered by this virus, most of the interviewed persons who expressed this consider it increased or particularly serious, but there are also voices expressing ***doubt about the real severity of the virus*** (S.C.), even in conditions where the interviews were conducted during the period when Romania, like most countries in the world, was under quarantine and lockdown measures, and the news presented by most media channels ***emphasized the presentation of suffering persons*** and those deceased as a result of contracting the virus.

An element that led to the accentuation of anguish and even panic among the population was the ***propagation of apocalyptic scenarios*** (A.J.), which included an exaggeratedly large number of deaths, an extreme contagion of the virus, almost impossible to counteract and avoid. The media insisted on presenting ***grim images*** (A.J.), including those of ***extreme visual violence*** - entire rooms full of black bags containing the corpses of those killed by Covid-19, in Italy, Spain, etc. These images could be associated in the collective mindset with similar images from horror movies, with ***post-apocalyptic scenarios***, where a pandemic reduces the planet's population to near complete annihilation. All these aspects induced in some of the interviewed persons the idea of a ***deliberate hyperbolization of the virus's severity*** by authorities or the media, in contrast with their ***own experience in contact with the virus*** or with persons who previously had the virus.

Another question mark regarding the infection rate was the lack of infected persons in the circle of acquaintances of the interviewed persons, which raised questions either about its virulence or ***the existence and severity of its symptomatology***. On the opposite end, there were interviewed persons who declared that they personally experienced infection with the virus, in a more or less severe form, among these being persons who consider that ***the severity of the virus's symptoms is exaggerated***, compared to ***their own experience of the disease***. However, there were also persons who ***required hospitalization*** - either the interviewee personally, or family members or acquaintances/close ones, or who even had deaths among their acquaintances.

There were persons who declared that a source of anguish - sometimes considered the most intense - is related to ***hospital conditions*** (A.M.C.) and the lack of medicines and sanitary materials, but also to ***poor care*** and even the ***impossibility of communication*** between the patient infected with Covid-19, hospitalized, and family. A high degree of anguish was manifested by persons in risk groups regarding severe forms of Covid-19 disease, whether it's elderly persons or those suffering from comorbidities. *The biggest imbalance appeared on the psychological side. [...] The stress was much greater than for a healthy person, because the disease itself is of an affective-emotional nature and I knew for sure that if I contracted this virus, the consequences could be much more drastic and, therefore, sometimes, imbalances appeared in my blood sugar and in my physical and mental state, due to the fear of not catching this virus and not ending up in the hospital (seeing and knowing the problems that are at the county hospitals and, respectively, at the county hospital), and I no longer had that assurance that I would be treated there and receive appropriate care, not necessarily for Coronavirus, but for diabetes, which needs to be more careful care* (G.G. - person with type I insulin-dependent diabetes). In the same direction, another person declares that one of the sources of anxiety is the possibility of contracting a disease other than Covid-19, which would necessitate ***contact with the hospital environment*** and, due to improper conditions in Romanian hospitals, to become infected with Coronavirus and develop a severe form of this disease. The subject even considers that ***the highest risk of infection is in the hospital environment***, for patients with other diseases or for medical staff. Hygiene conditions, inefficient triage, lack of sanitary and protective equipment make the interviewed subject not trust in the possibility of the healthcare system to effectively treat patients ill with Covid-19 or, at least, not to subject patients to ***additional infection risks***, preferring to ***avoid at all costs*** contact with the hospital environment and even with the healthcare environment, even in the hypothesis of contracting a mild form of the disease:

First of all, I can say that I was afraid of not getting injured or feeling ill and ending up in the hospital, where there were very high chances of getting infected and, due to the panic in the hospital and the scared staff, not receiving appropriate and complete care. And, as we well know, the medical system in Romania is not very well set up (B.A.G.).

The interviewed persons generally declared that the ***fear of infection*** appeared when they learned that persons close to them had contracted the virus and that it manifests in quite severe or even particularly severe forms. Relating to others induced forms of fear, anguish, or even anxiety. In some situations, fear is mentioned as being explicitly manifested in relation to more vulnerable persons in one's own family (A.A.), (D.A.B.) or among close ones. A ***stoic attitude*** is signaled even in ***elderly persons***, who accept with some serenity the prospect of possible illness and even loss of their own life, but manifest feelings of fear for the life and health of their loved ones: *I have a great fear of the pandemic for children, grandchildren, because they are young, their life is ahead. About myself no fear, I am old, I will die anyway either now or later (S.A.). The suffering of others hurts more deeply than my own suffering* (D.S.).

In the case of some interviewees, the ***first news*** about the spread of the virus and the emergence of the pandemic produced ***panic***, later declaring that they adopted a coping strategy - in the sense of accepting the disease as an ***inevitable reality*** that will accompany us in the long term, even after the end of the lockdown period (N.N.1). Thus, a reason for anxiety is ***the impossibility of predicting the duration of the pandemic situation*** - both in general, until returning to a ***post-pandemic „normal"***, and in particular, ***during the lockdown period*** which, once prolonged, can have consequences regarding the ***budgetary resources*** of the person and family, health status, etc. *They are afraid that the quarantine will be extended for an indefinite period and they will not have resources to support their family.* (A.O.).

Also, ***fear for one's own health condition*** is present in the interviewed persons (D.A.B.), (D.M.C.). Stress caused by ***prolonged isolation*** (*for two months*) has also caused other health problems - related, but not necessarily (D.A.B.). Among the symptoms associated with stress and anxiety were mentioned ***fatigue, increased nervousness, and irritability***: *I am always tired, although I don't do much, also, I get angry very quickly over trifles. I get angry quickly and I can't concentrate on absolutely anything, I can't rest properly and I stress a lot* (S.R.).

The main sources of anxiety highlighted were related to the ***interruption of daily activities***, quarantine (L.B.), the fact that people were forced to stay ***away from loved ones*** (D.A.B.) - which is, in our understanding, ***an extension of the idea of***

social distancing, from ***limiting physical proximity*** to ***limiting social communication***. *Lack of freedom, communication, and the need for people* (P.I.3) are considered the main sources of population anguish and frustration.

Situations were presented of elderly persons who, despite the prohibition of leaving home[3], were caught taking walks and/or trips that they did not make before the state of emergency. *Many did not respect this measure. At least in my neighborhood, I see dozens of elderly people walking daily, who before the pandemic did not go out* (B.R.). We attribute this attitude to the development, by the respective persons, of coping mechanisms to the pandemic situation, in which ***the feeling of freedom is more important than that of safety***. This may be especially true for elderly persons living alone, especially those who have deficient skills in using electronic means of communication and who, for example, display themselves outside the home to communicate their own existence to others, but also to become, perhaps involuntarily, aware that their situation is still acceptable. Of course, at least in the case of some persons who made fewer trips before the pandemic, intensifying them after the declaration

[3] The ban on leaving home was valid for the entire population of the country, not just for those in quarantined localities, the exception to this rule being current needs, supplies, travel to work, care for sick people, etc., and could only be carried out based on a declaration on one's own responsibility regarding the destination, route and duration of the trip. For the elderly, time intervals were established, during which an almost complete restriction on travel was in force.

of the state of emergency, it may be a matter of ***the need for self-supply***, when close persons, who usually provided their current supply, were perhaps in quarantine, in other isolated localities, or isolated in their own home, for medical reasons, or in quarantine instituted for certain socio-professional categories.

Awareness of the severity of the virus generated states of anxiety and panic, which we attribute to the awareness of risks (A.A.) for one's own health and ***the appearance of radical changes in lifestyle***. The two components lead us to the idea of awareness that people live in an increasingly deeply medicalized risk society. The virus is considered to be much stronger than we choose to perceive it (A.A.). We note that ***the perceived severity of the public health problem*** raised by Covid-19 infection is considered to be a choice and that the interviewee (A.A.) considers that, for various reasons specific to each person, the individual chooses to perceive the virus as less serious than it is in reality, despite messages from the media and warnings from national and international authorities. The same effect can be thought of in the opposite direction, of a hyperbolized perception of the virus's severity, which can even lead to a ***state of despair*** (A. N.) of the population and which, on the other hand, can help the individual develop compliance with measures proposed by health authorities, which will later be contested as exaggerated. Another factor that generated panic among the population was ***the unexpected appearance and very rapid spread of the virus*** (D.A.B.). The interviewed persons express their concern about how and to what extent the current pandemic will affect their future - and not just from a medical point of view (D.A.B). Some even appreciate that mass immunization represents a solution for eliminating or diminishing the long-term effects of the pandemic (L.B). The interviewed persons showed their concern about the possible deterioration of the economic situation and the emergence of a crisis (A.B.).

Another feeling towards the situation caused by the pandemic, described by the interviewed persons, is that of ***revolt***: *I felt the need to protect my own and I knew I couldn't do this alone, and that revolted me* (S.P.). A special mention of the category of those who declared that they felt feelings of revolt is related to the restriction and/or limitation of access to medical services, other than those intended for the care of persons infected with Covid-19: *I was revolted by the fact that we were not allowed to go to hospitals for a consultation or routine analyses* (M.T.). *This crisis has caused the appointments I had with various doctors to be postponed and, thus, I don't know exactly what the situation is regarding my health status* (A.N.).

Some respondents, especially those under 25 years old, state that they did not experience anguish due to the danger of possible illness, relying on information circulating in the public environment at that time, according to which the people most predisposed to infection are the elderly and those with comorbidities. Analyzing the statements of one of the interviewed persons (S.D.B.), who declares that they followed quarantine measures, we consider that they did not construct an image of the possibility of their own infection - a fact that could have led to ***ignoring infection prevention measures***. Some interviewed persons declared that ***they became aware of the risks caused by the pandemic later***, with the establishment of the state of emergency (C.M.C.), (L.C.), initially not taking seriously the authorities' warnings and necessary preventive measures (A.B.). *It was a mixture of feelings. Initially, I mocked it, believing it was just a lie or a situation to scare us* (I.A.B.). Other persons, on the contrary (N.N.1), as they found that ***the measures taken by authorities were not credible*** from their point of view, gave up applying them, going as far as no longer believing in the existence of the virus or, at least, in the severity of its threat.

Another major cause of the installation of anguish among the population is considered to be the ***lack of communication*** (A.B.), both between citizens - aggravated by ***inefficient public communication*** - and by the ***large number of fake news***, which makes public communication little credible and/or wrongly perceived by the population. Opinions were also recorded according to which ***the severity of the infection is exaggerated***, persons presenting mild symptoms that would not normally have required medical intervention appealed to emergency medical services - on the one hand, panicking and accentuating the panic of those around them and, on the other hand, endangering the health system's response capacity to truly emergency situations (D.B.).

Indeed, we cannot help but notice that medical intervention protocols have been modified, which in the first months after the declaration of the pandemic required the use of the ***isolette***, and later, after a few months, required the person declared positive to travel alone or with the help of public transport to the emergency hospital, or just to self-isolate at home, without resorting to a medical consultation. ***The image of the isolette*** remained in the collective mindset as a symbol of this pandemic, along with ***the mask*** and ***social distancing***, and created a new social fear - ***fear of the isolette***, correlated with and extended to ***fear of doctors*** and the health system. In other words, the isolette will remain in the collective mindset a phrase similar to the classic "bogeyman" (see images of people wearing beaked masks during plague pandemics - hence the name "undertakers", which in popular language designates people who gather the dead).

Those who express anguish hierarchize it from minor states of ***fear*** towards the phenomenon, to real states of "***horror***" towards the danger represented by the virus, especially in the context of other systemic crises affecting the population (from Moldova, in the case of the respondent who made the quoted statement). This pandemic is perceived as an "attack" both on citizens' freedom and on public health. We correlate this statement, referring to comparing the pandemic with an attack, with other responses from the same interviewee, who describe the virus as a biological weapon in the hands of enemies of humanity.

Once panic set in, which is perceived as a product of misinformation and fake news, many felt ***the need to stock up*** on medicines and food, which later proved to be unnecessary (L.C.), but this creation of additional personal stocks ***accentuated panic***, registering a real contagion effect related to the state of panic. In fact, in addition to the Coronavirus pandemic, whose origin, dimension, and effects were partially unknown - and remained quite little known or, at least, controversial at the time of this study -, the population faced an ***undeclared epidemic of panic***, which affected the ***mental health of the population*** to an equal or even greater extent than the effects of Covid-19 infection, except for severe and very severe cases. Although not declared pandemic, because the transmission of panic is not documented as being community-based, ***the general state of anguish and panic of the population*** had effects that have not yet been highlighted and measured, but which, in our opinion, have ***accentuated the medicalization of society*** and the ***dependence on a therapeutic act*** - whether we are talking about a medical, psychological, social or spiritual one.

An additional element that strengthened the state of panic is represented by the reminiscences existing in collective memory regarding more or less close historical periods, which appeared after wars or during dictatorships such as the communist one, in which the lack of basic necessities - including food - was chronic and, therefore, creating surplus stocks had become a habit, taking the form of a survival culture. *Many people, even I often remember from the times of the U.S.S.R., when goods were often missing from store shelves. Other people fear the repetition of numerous crises, like those from previous years, when for a certain category of products the price could suddenly increase* (A.O.).

Another element generating panic was the ***aspect of hygiene***. One of the interviewed persons showed that, due to the panic that gripped them, they took ***exaggerated protective measures***, which even put their life in danger (L.C.), disinfecting large surfaces with substances that can be toxic, this being done in the absence of adequate disinfectants on the market. One of the interviewed persons showed that they felt *condemned* by this pandemic: *I felt that I would be condemned and that this is a disaster for all people* (N.N.3). ***The feeling of being condemned to suffering*** was strengthened by the abundance of news from the media regarding the pandemic and their contrariety, as well as by the panicked behavior of a large part of the population. The obligation to stay at home and the transformation of this necessity into an obligation - and, at the same time, into an official public policy - strengthened the interviewed person's conviction that the crisis situation will be a long-lasting one: *it will last forever and we will be forced more and more to stay at home* (N.N.3).

The lack of perspective regarding ***the return to the situation of normality*** is seen as ***an incarceration in one's own home***, without being about guilt, and this is perceived in the case of the mentioned person as a personal and collective misfortune at the same time.

Another problem touched upon by the same interviewed subject is ***the transfer of educational interactions to the virtual environment - the virtualization of social space*** (n.n.) - emphasizing online education, a system for which both teachers and students/pupils were taken completely by surprise, being totally unprepared. According to the interviewed person, this ***limits both the quality of education*** and ***the satisfaction related to the teaching act***, for both teachers and its beneficiaries: *The moment I started the virtual courses, I realized that my health is put into question, because I spend hours in front of the computer and, after 8 hours of looking at the laptop screen, I looked in the mirror and saw dark circles and tired "zombie" eyes. I tried to go out on the balcony to look at the world, but I realized that the world is no longer outside, I was only looking at the birds* (N.N.3).

The approach to the pandemic has made many confront the fear of death and, of course, there were people who even prepared for imminent death. A simple feverish state leads, under the effect of panic, automatically to thoughts of infection, and this generates anguish, through anticipation of one's own death, but also of the effects it will have on loved ones. People who exercise, during the pandemic period, ***duties that involve direct contact with the public***, experience additional anguish, related to the fact that they could ***themselves be the source of infection for their clients*** and, implicitly, the cause of their possible death.

There are also people who declared that ***they did not personally experience anguish or anxiety*** in correlation with the Coronavirus pandemic. Some of these, however, showed that, although they did not experience these states personally - for example, due to a stable financial situation - they knew people who experienced them and were affected by these states (P.I.2). We consider it worth mentioning that interviewees from the Republic of Moldova showed that, in general, the perception regarding the severity of the disease and the seriousness of respecting quarantine measures was more pronounced in Romania, where the level of anxiety was also higher than in the Republic of Moldova, the differences could be attributed to differences in quality of life and lifestyle between the inhabitants of the two countries, but also to the general tendency of the population from the Republic of Moldova to approach a more spartan conduct, more inclined to minimize the negative effects of a situation and, we believe, to reduce the level of medicalization of society, compared to the conduct of the population from Romania.

III.8. Impact of news about the pandemic

The interviewed persons express their point of view regarding ***the impact of news related to the pandemic***, this being ***mostly negative***, but there are also people who showed that ***they were not extremely affected***: *I can't say that they had a bad impact on me, but at one point I really got tired of these news and messages from the media, everywhere you heard* *only about Coronavirus* (P.I.2). There are also voices that emphasize the positive role that the media should play in such a situation - to encourage the population to respect the necessary protective measures and, at the same time, to inform the population about ***possible deviations from normality*** that may appear during a crisis period, and to point out people who try, through illegitimate manners, to create advantages for themselves during the crisis period, taking advantage of it and exploiting possible limits of the public system: *The media is considered the third political power in a democratic state, thus, it influences to a very large percentage; it focuses on protective measures and highlights the idea of protecting ourselves, by the fact that we must stay at home as much as possible and respect the rest of the imposed measures. It also discovers some irregularities, which are not so obvious for the rest of the population, thus drawing attention to them, being subjected to our attention* (A.C.).

III.9. Perceived effects of the pandemic

Positive effects: Some interviewed persons declared that the Coronavirus pandemic also had ***beneficial effects***, including ***appreciation of important things in life*** and time spent with loved ones (D.A.B.), (I.A.B.), (A.S.B.). Another important thing, considered to be a positive effect of going through this pandemic, is, according to one of the respondents: *I started to love life more* (L.C.). ***Acute awareness of the fear of death*** makes other elements of dissatisfaction, related to living standards, quality of life, etc., no longer viewed with such importance, compared to ***the value of life itself***. Among the interviewed persons, there are some respondents who appreciate ***the positive role of the pandemic*** in the social construction of responsibility for one's own health, towards others and towards the environment: *[the pandemic] clearly had a beneficial role. Thus, in a relatively short time, a collective responsibility towards hygiene measures was consolidated. At the same time, stopping and limiting some forms of industry had a visible beneficial impact on the environment (N.N.4).* In the same direction, another respondent states that: *Perhaps our planet needed a moment of solitude, in which to recharge its batteries, to regenerate through its own forces. People are very negligent with nature! Waste thrown into waters, air choked by smoke produced by cars and factories, packaging forgotten on streets and parks have made the environment in which we live become polluted. This isolation has become an ideal opportunity to put a stop to our harmful habits* (I.E.).

People who appreciated the existence of beneficial effects of lockdown referred, among other things, to the development of a ***capacity for self-control over daily routines***, more efficient organization of activities, and adoption of a responsible lifestyle: *I learned to be much more organized than I was before the appearance of this pandemic and I arranged my days so that there is progress in my life, and not a regression. [...] The only hobby I frequented abusively was cooking, I took care,* *however, this time, to use much healthier foods, to be careful what I eat, how much I eat, so that at the end of isolation I don't cry* (A.M.).

Negative effects: Among the negative effects of the pandemic were reported: ***depreciation of long-term health condition*** of many people (see sequelae, length of convalescence period, ***sedentary lifestyle*** imposed by the pandemic - which predisposes to a decrease in the immune system and vitality of the organism), but also ***loss of human lives***. The lack of movement is also brought into discussion - at least that performed outdoors (B.S.A.): *one goes crazy just staying at home, they should at least be allowed to go out to the field, to the park* (A.B.). The interviewed person shows that he himself seeks to diminish the effects of the prohibition to leave his own home, dedicating himself to learning activities, relaxation, and practicing meditation (A.B.). The risks of ***mental disorders*** are underlined in the context in which the diminution of practicing hobbies and, especially, outdoor activities is discussed: *Honestly, I would have liked to have read more physical books and not those on the laptop, because I don't like them and, at the same time, I would have liked to have the possibility to walk more outside; staying at home is not good for the brain, nor for the body, nor for the psyche* (A.M.).

The interviewed persons express hope that the experience of the pandemic will also have ***transformative effects***, in the sense of changing people's attitude / behavior towards the environment, and not only (L.B).

Even the ***risk of death*** not directly due to Covid-19 illness, but to other collateral causes, such as ***lack of access to health services, lack of basic care*** for the elderly and, why not, ***severe depreciation of the mental condition*** of persons belonging to vulnerable categories is brought into discussion: *This crisis makes the elderly stay locked in the house and perish* (P.I.2).

In addition to the mentioned effects on public health, those on the economic environment are also brought into discussion, as well as ***the possibility of a major economic crisis*** in the post-pandemic period (D.A.B.). There were people who declared that among their acquaintances there are people who ***lost their jobs*** during the pandemic or are in temporary unemployment, thus bringing into discussion a ***severe diminution of their financial resources*** (P.I.2).

While respondents show that infection risks are higher among the elderly population - as was appreciated at the time of the interviews -, regarding negative economic effects, these are reflected especially on people of active age and especially on young people. ***The risk of social marginalization*** (A.B.) of various categories of population affected by both the health crisis and the economic one is also perceived, associated with the lack or reduction of material resources - especially against the background of the perception of lack of resources, generally at the level of society, but especially at the state level, to overcome the economic and social crisis, which is perceived as severe.

The negative impact on the population was also felt through the ***restriction of the right to work*** and the limitation of the right to free movement, a situation described by one of the interviewed persons as generating ***a state of helplessness*** (D.M.C.).

The massive presence of ***armed law enforcement forces*** (I.A.B.) on the streets, during the beginning of the self-isolation period, contributed to increasing the population's anguish, having a negative impact on public trust in authorities, who were seeking to impose quarantine measures, by increasing law enforcement forces and through measures meant to create ***the impression of a militarized control*** of the situation, to the detriment of streamlining public communication.

Another element perceived as generating anxiety and frustration was the ***obligation of self-quarantine*** (D.B.) for those who carried out their professional activity in medical, social or medico-social care institutions. This self-quarantine of medical personnel, but also of those in social assistance or other professions related to care - not necessarily of persons infected with this virus - was much more severe than the isolation measures imposed on the general population and prohibited any form of leaving the home or isolation residence, as well as contact with any person, including family members. This situation was often perceived as a form of deprivation of liberty (L.C.) and, implicitly, of ***violation of fundamental rights***. Also in the context of depriving citizens of exercising fundamental rights, the ***deprivation of treatment*** for persons suffering from various pathologies - other than Covid-19 - can be included, due to the transformation of most hospitals into Covid or Covid-support hospitals and the limitation, through ***military ordinances*** in force, of carrying out medical acts considered non-essential. However, the list of medical acts considered non-essential sometimes included therapies which, although they did not involve emergency intervention, could prove life-saving later or could prevent irreversible deterioration of patients' quality of life.

Another effect, perceived at the level of the ***economic environment*** this time, is ***the imminence of bankruptcy*** for many small and medium businesses, but possibly also for some large companies, caused by temporary closure of activity, lack of liquidity, inability to pay, etc. Some of the respondents declared that they felt ***compassion for the affected business representatives***, but also for the employees of those companies: *[I felt] pity, extremely many businesses could go bankrupt* (G.S.).

III.10. Credibility of information sources and infodemic

Respondents indicate that ***available sources of information***, especially mass media, ***are generally not credible*** - they are *manipulative* (L.B.) - and therefore, subjects cannot inform themselves completely, correctly, and especially credibly from these sources. The increase in the number of ***fake news*** has also been a source of stress and anxiety for citizens, with interviewed persons showing that they felt threatened by the explosion in the number of false news (A.B.). ***The abundance of false news*** related to the pandemic is criticized by respondents, being attributed to the desire of the press *to overwhelm with so much information* (A.B.).

There are people who have drawn attention to the fact that, in such situations, such as those in which the state of emergency is active, taking measures to restrict freedom of expression - with the aim of controlling false and, especially, alarmist news - is welcome: *What affected me the most was the freedom of the media. The media had a freedom to express a rather alarming opinion and creates fear and panic among the population. I think the media should have been controlled a little in this period, from the point of view of some dramatic news... a much greater dramatism was created than the situation itself, although this virus is quite dangerous and we must treat it as such* (G.G. - person with type I insulin-dependent diabetes).

III.11. Perception of the post-pandemic period

Many of the interviewed persons consider that, sooner or later, *the situation will return to normal* (D.M.C.) from an epidemiological and public health perspective, with many of them being more concerned about the evolution of the economic and social situation. ***The hope of returning to normalcy*** represents, from our point of view, an

attempt to humanize the pandemic experience, especially as one of the interviewed persons declares that during the pandemic period they carried out a series of daily activities in their own household, activities that involved contact with nature: *Living in the countryside, I take care of the household, of animals, I plant trees, spring being the season when there is the most work, I don't get bored* (D.C.). However, the same person feels the need to express that, immediately after the relaxation of quarantine, they intend to interact with their loved one through a walk in nature together[4].

Another idea, which also leads to the construct of ***post-pandemic normality***, is that of returning to freedom of movement, at least within the locality of residence, without the risk of being stopped by the Police and interrogated about destination, duration of travel, etc.: *I will be able to go where I want in the city, without being afraid if the police would stop me* (N.I.). As we mentioned earlier, the ***humanization of the everyday life*** is the key desideratum for post-pandemic society. Within this humanization of the everyday, a particularly important element is the ***elimination of fear*** from the foreground of relating to social life.

Practically, the pandemic is also seen as an ***invitation to responsibility*** - both to the immediate responsibilization of each individual, and to the long-term responsibility of individuals, but also of

[4] All interviews were conducted during the lockdown period in Romania. As such, the interviewee expresses a desire for when these measures will be relaxed.

communities. Immediate effects, such as ***increasing the level of hygiene of individuals***, but also of communities, ***reducing some emissions with polluting effect*** - by limiting vehicle traffic, for example - have constituted examples of responsible attitudes or responsibilizing measures, which affect the population in the short term, but which can become long-term social habitus. In their absence, even if the pandemic will end, their effects could last much longer (T.C.). Post-pandemic society is seen by some respondents as one of ***increased responsibility installed in the collective mindset*** (for example, in the form of daily mask-wearing): *I see the future with many people with masks on the street, but more careful than ever. [...] There will always be someone who gets sick* (N.N.1). This responsibility towards others and towards one's own health condition is, in our opinion, a marker of the acceptance of post-pandemic society as a risk society and of the accentuation of the medicalization of society, in the sense that the human condition will be perceived, itself, as a treatable disorder, and the encounter with the Other will be perceived in the sense of encountering danger - in this case, with a possible source of infection. *Unfortunately, we will avoid each other. We will all be a danger to all* (B.R.). Even if it was not emphasized as such in the responses of the interviewed persons, ***the depreciation of the relationship with the other*** through the deculturalized and deculturalizing presence of the mask, if it becomes a defining element of post-pandemic society, will be able to destructure sociability to a point where ***the singularity of individuals*** can no longer be compensated through communication processes, thus accentuating the tendency towards an ***individualistic society*** and, ultimately, a selfish society. Even if wearing a mask is justified by medical reasons, it cannot be easily separated in the collective mindset from the symbol of the mask, as a factor of hiding the person and personality in front of an Other, with whom we limit communication to the maximum, because we are afraid. A de-solidarized society generates ***an anguish of the presence of the other*** as a possible source of infection and which goes as far as to refuse its presence in the immediate vicinity, the subject itself being able to become the source of anguish, related to the depreciation of quality of life in correlation with the state of health. Life in a medicalized society can at some point be a flight from any risks which, reaching paroxysm, can eliminate the subjective quality of life for the sake of a so-called objective quality, measured in an apparent state of health, translated by the absence of an acute infection, but with the permanent presence of social or psychological dysfunctions.

There are also opinions according to which ***returning to "normal" will be impossible***, the virus will continue to exist, as other dangerous viruses exist, and ***society will get used to living with the threat of new pandemic waves***, which will bring new lockdown measures and, at the same time, the population will have to be more responsible in terms of respecting hygiene measures, including those specific to these pandemics - wearing masks, gloves, physical but also social distancing, etc.: *I don't think we will return so soon to life before, no matter how much we want to... It is a virus that we will carry, most certainly, for years, just as HIV exists, just as Tuberculosis exists, Coronavirus will also exist, it will be present among us, maybe it will not affect such a considerable number of people anymore, but I think we never return to the days where we live quietly and happily, without having the fear that we will get sick again, that we will be forced to stay at home, that this quarantine will return, this period of total pause. [...] We have no way to eliminate the past, to return to a point where you can't. This is the course of life, this is how it must continue. There are good parts, and bad parts, and we must move forward. The fear that this virus will invade the whole world again exists and will remain forever, at least among the next two or three generations... or until the point where a miraculous treatment for all humanity on the globe will be discovered* (A.M.).

Those who affirm that life in the post-pandemic period will be different or even radically different from that before the appearance of the first signs of the pandemic, consider that it takes time for the population to get used to the necessary measures and, due to this time and anticipatory socialization, correlated with physical distancing measures, which also include real social distancing, the style and way of life will be different, but the population will adapt, sooner or later: *The sooner we get used to the new way of life, the sooner this new way of life will seem normal to us* (T.T.).

III.12. Post-pandemic immediateness

A widely held opinion among the interviewed persons is that the exit from lockdown will have to prioritize ***the recovery of sociability***. Social distancing measures, although aimed at creating a safety space around the person to reduce the possibility of infection, bring restrictions regarding sociability or, more precisely, ***the social rituals*** to which individuals are accustomed, radically changing them: handshaking, hugging, kissing on the cheek - are all gestures with social ritual value that are not only forbidden, but also acquire ***a value with social risk***. Even when we are not talking about strict quarantine and movement is possible in certain areas, even with a declaration, the number of people in a group, the number of people who can participate in an event, the duration of meetings, and especially the performance of these social rituals with value of expressing solidarity and sociability were limited. Their recovery is seen as ***a recovery of the essential***. One of the interviewed subjects shows that the first thing they will do after the restrictions or, at least, the lockdown ends will be *to see my acquaintances, my circle of friends again. These are the important things* (C.C.). Of course, in their statement, ***sociability*** transpires ***as a fundamental ethical and cultural value*** for the subject and which, certainly, is in consonance with the point of view of many other individuals, including some of those interviewed, who consider communication with acquaintances, with the circle of friends, with close ones, in general, as being an element of utmost importance for their subjective well-being. The desire for normality is expressed in the form of returning to everyday naturalness, part of life that was, perhaps, the most affected during the pandemic period: *I will walk with my loved one in the park* (D.C.).

III.13. The transfer of daily activities to online (virtualization of social space)

Some interviewed persons showed that ***the obligation to work from home*** produced ***radical changes in their work schedule***. This is valid in several professional areas, where companies or institutions have chosen to switch to working from home / online activity. A significant case, in which all activity was transferred online, is that of ***education***, where from the beginning of the pandemic until the end of the state of emergency, and even after its end, the activity was conducted exclusively online, which ***significantly disrupted both the work schedule and lifestyle*** - of both students and teachers (B.S.A.*)*. *Unfortunately, I had countless ups and downs. If at first my whole schedule was turned upside down, I lost the notion of days, time and my usual routine, I had to force myself to return to the initial period and reorganize myself* (A.M.). Conducting online educational activity is hampered by the lack of feedback from students, but also by the relative novelty of this teaching/learning style. The lack of direct and personal interactions between teachers and students constitutes another reason for dissatisfaction with online education, considered for this reason to be much more difficult (B.S.A.). In this context, some people show that this transition to online is ***a source of discomfort***, which can lead to various forms of migraines and even alteration of health: *The fact that I cannot carry out my activities as usual is harmful to me, because I am forced to continue my studies in the online environment, which is very difficult, because I spend too much time in front of the laptop screen and unbearable eye and head pains appear.* (S.D.)

The massive virtualization of social interactions - in this case educational ones - during the lockdown period took many by surprise, making it so that in the first period, when all courses were transitioned online, they were not at the best educational standards, as students are accustomed to for day courses, for which online study mechanisms have not yet been correctly and completely established: *I was no longer able to understand the courses, the teachers taught 90% in Spanish and not in English, as they used to do at the faculty, and secondly it was difficult for me to keep up with everyone, because the internet was freezing, the teachers were speaking quite fast, colleagues even faster and, at some moments, some colleagues were using the Galician dialect, which was a bit complicated for me, to understand word by word* [5](A.M.).

---

[5] The interview belongs to a student who, at the time of the interview, was studying at a university in Spain.

The transition to the virtual environment of many economic, but also educational activities, is seen ***ambivalently,*** on one hand as ***saving time and effort*** for students, teachers, employees, etc., on the other hand ***it requires an adaptation*** of professional activities and ***behaviors*** to the virtual environment: *At first it seemed more comfortable to me, because I didn't have to travel to the faculty by bus and between stations anymore, then I realized that this technique of teaching in the online environment and not at the faculty is not as pleasant. For example, one of the biggest difficulties I encountered from the beginning was the fact that, if we were presented with a certain exercise on the computer that we had to do at the same time as the teacher, and we only had two laptops available, we decided to use one of them to observe what the teacher does, and on the other to work* (A.M.).

A ***positive effect of the virtualization of social space*** is ***the possibility of communication*** with people at a distance, with whom subjects otherwise keep in touch less frequently when activity is predominantly conducted in the physical environment. Some interviewed persons showed that ***they keep in touch with their loved ones*** through ***social networks***, because it is impossible for them to meet physically, due to imposed isolation and self-isolation measures (A.S.B.). In such lockdown periods, when socializing actions are transferred to the online environment, ***physical distances are suppressed by online communication***, physical proximity no longer being necessary for maintaining or rediscovering relationships: *I talked to all the people, with whom I probably didn't communicate so often before or with whom I never talked so much* (A.M.).

III.14. Protective measures and approaches to the pandemic situation proposed by the interviewed persons

In accordance with some measures publicly imposed by authorities, the interviewed persons also emphasize ***the importance of preventive testing*** for detecting infected but asymptomatic persons, ***the availability of disinfectant and hygiene products***[6], and the drastic limitation of public meetings and manifestations (B.S.A.). There were voices indicating the need to improve ***triage measures*** at the entrance to hospitals or care centers (B.R.). Some interviewed persons recommend to everyone ***to maintain calm and lucidity*** (D.M.C.), in order to more easily overcome the problems that have arisen during this period.

Religious experience, as well as ***daily routines***, are other measures that individuals consider useful for ***reducing the psychological effects of the pandemic***, which can be associated with methods for reducing the biological effects of virus transmission. Subjects have exposed that they resort to prayer, but also to

[6] At the time of the research, these measures were already routinely implemented. Every public place provides disinfectants to people. However, at the time of the interview, there was a shortage of disinfectants in Romania, including being unavailable on the market.

daily routine (B.R.), others discover or deepen the practice of hobbies or carry out activities that occupy their time: reading, watching movies, series, continuing educational or professional activity online and deepening relationships with friends, family or acquaintances through online or telephone communication means.

An interesting suggestion for overcoming stress during this period is to note thoughts, ideas, experiences lived during the pandemic in the form of a ***journal/diary:*** *what bothered me I wrote down on paper and so I can say that I did not let myself be brought to my knees by this fear* (I.E.).

Another solution for overcoming stress and anxiety caused by the pandemic is ***the presence of pets***: ***Also, the time spent with pets helped me to view the situation with optimism and to enjoy every moment of life*** (B.A.).

III.15. Conspiracy theories regarding the pandemic and Coronavirus

There are people who declare that ***they are convinced of the non-existence of the SARS-COV-2 virus*** and the disease it generates, and the "so-called pandemic", in their view, is actually a ***global conspiracy***: *it's nothing but a global conspiracy. It's a total invention, this virus doesn't exist* (V.C.). Consistent with their own point of view, the person shows that ***they refuse to comply with the protective measures*** imposed by authorities and violate quarantine. In public debate, especially in alternative media and on social networks, accepting or denying the existence of the virus becomes a matter of faith expressed through phrases like "I believe / don't believe in Covid". This attitude towards Covid-19 is connected with ***trust in science***, in authorities, and in the various sources of information to which the individual has access.

The existence of ***inexplicable elements or incorrectly explained by authorities, contradictory messages***, and radical preventive measures that seem to be overestimated compared to the situation perceived in the immediate vicinity of people and which is in contrast with that presented by the media, makes those who, for various reasons, show distrust in authorities, adhere to negationist views, to conspiracy theories that question the existence of the virus or, on the contrary, place it in the category of ***weapons of mass destruction***, used by ***occult forces*** for ***population reduction***, etc.

Among the interviewed persons, there are also some who consider the Covid-19 virus *a biological weapon developed to reduce the number of people in the world* (L.C.). The interviewed person reaches this conclusion precisely because of the way the virus spreads, which allows it *to spread its traces very quickly and thus endanger the entire universe* (L.C.). Indeed, a widespread tendency is observable - among those who are adherents of various conspiracy theories regarding this virus - to hyperbolize the spread of the virus to give weight to their own statements, with global spread being extrapolated to the level of the entire universe. The idea that ***this***

virus is of synthetic origin is widespread, being maintained including by statements of political officials, influential people in the media, but also representatives of the medical world.

Another approach, which may be connected with conspiracy theory, is that the measures taken by governments do not actually aim to reduce the number of infected people, but to generate and exacerbate the already existing crisis at the economic and social level (L.C.). The idea of the virus's appearance, but also of the crisis generated by the pandemic in general, is attributed by some interviewed persons to the existence of an ***unconventional war*** - either between the great powers of the world, or between supranational organizations, which use biological terrorism and biological weapons, possibly out of control, to generate panic and create economic, political, and even military instability at a global level. This position is sometimes accentuated by ***the idea of reducing the population number***, a common idea in many conspiracy theories, but there are also answers that emphasize the economic impact of this crisis, which generates economic and political instability, potentially leading even to ***a New World Order*** (D.S.), to a rearrangement of the military, but especially economic balance, at a global level: *this virus was designed to affect the world economy* (P.I.4).

Without constituting a subject of a proper conspiracy theory, many interviewed persons have emphasized ***the negative role of mass media***, both classical and internet, in creating a state of panic.

Many consider that ***panic-generating news*** was ***intentionally transmitted*** for this purpose: *Those who represent the mass media, the people behind the monitors have intentionally instilled fear in people, in my opinion* (N.G.). ***The contradictory nature of news*** presented in mass media and, especially, in new media has bewildered public opinion, making ***the infodemic*** - or the epidemic of fake news - sometimes considered more serious than the actual pandemic. Censorship of communication on various online channels, under the pretext of "violating community standards", was applied even to voices from the sphere of science, but also politics, the case of censoring Donald Trump's speeches being eloquent. Although the measure of ***censoring messages*** that generate anarchy and panic is beneficial to a certain point and absolutely necessary to achieve ***social balance*** in a period of crisis, large sectors of the population have felt the return of censorship, which especially citizens from former communist countries associate with left or right ***dictatorships***. *As far as I'm concerned, uncertainty speaks for itself, because I don't know many things about this pandemic and in the mass media I see many different opinions, and these certainly cause me states of anxiety* (N.G.).

III.16. Perception on the pandemic

Regarding the general perception of the pandemic, as experienced by the interviewed persons, it refers to aspects such as severity, impact, emotional reference, changes in lifestyle, all these elements being included in other specific categories or subcategories. Within this category, we have retained those references to perceptions of subjects that could not be included in other categories, but which we cannot ignore, due to the informational load regarding how subjects create meaning about the situation they are facing. We notice an interpretative drift of some concepts that subjects perceive as ambivalent, regarding their relation to the pandemic as a life situation - beyond the psychological states created, perceived or estimated effects, etc.

A first such subjective perception of the pandemic concerns its ***violent and unexpected character***. What interests us, from the perspective of this category, is ***the personification of the pandemic as an almost anthropologized force***, which seems to be credited with its own will and mode of action, reminiscent of the personification of natural forces in the form of benevolent or malevolent gods or demons: *I perceived it as a storm coming from nothingness, that swooped down on Earth* (I.E.). This ***subjectivized autonomy*** of the virus makes the subject relate to it not as a random genetic event (genetic mutation in the viral body), but as an energy or force that makes its presence and potency felt, seeming to have a purpose - obvious or imperceptible - and against which a ***magical/mystical approach*** or, at least, an animistic one is necessary. In general, people who, consciously or not, have this tendency to totemize such subjects, will be more susceptible to ***rejecting the scientific approach*** (genome sequencing, creating a vaccine through synthetic biology, etc.). Such an attitude can be understood as a "re-enchantment of the world", as a reaction to the ***apparent failure of technology***. In a world where hidden and intentional meanings are attributed to such events, scientific neutrality is "sanctioned" as being the result of a "plandemic" - that is, of an occult intentionality, thus making room for conspiracy theories. However, in this context, we must mention that the interviewed subject quoted above, although somewhat personifying the appearance of the virus, does not refer to elements that could lead to a synthetic theory of it, maintaining himself in the register of anthropomorphization of natural elements and a magical, even shamanic battle with this invisible force: *I got stuck in a process of fear, having other chronic diseases, but for a short time, because I realized that I have nowhere to run from this situation and I faced reality, [...] and so I can say that I did not let myself be brought to my knees by this fear* (I.E.).

The pandemic experience allows the person to ***reflect on the meaning of life*** and possible causes of human beings' departure from simplicity and naturalness, returning to these meaning ***recovering the value of life***: *Being blinded by the desire to gain money, power, I realized that we have neglected the essential aspects of life, namely self-knowledge and health, so I consider that the most important action we can undertake in order to alleviate suffering is to take care of ourselves and follow our instinct* (I.E.).

In parallel with the animist-type attitude, another subjective perception of the pandemic is of a ***teleological*** nature - all life events, including this pandemic, ***have a purpose that may or may not be decrypted***. The existence of a profound purpose, sometimes even evolutionary of events - or at least the belief in this existence - helps the person psychologically cope with anxiety generated by situations perceived as absurd and which the individual cannot easily oppose, such as: anguish in the face of death or terrible suffering, anguish in the face of loneliness and the impossibility or limitation of communication with others, the limitation of capacity and freedom of action, etc. All these anguishes, in the face of various limits of the human condition, have been evoked by this pandemic, and the reaction of attributing a purpose to it, along with an intention, helps people who adhere to belief in a Universe animated by unseen forces - Divinity, subtle presences, demonic - to give meaning to events and thus free themselves from the burden of their own ineffectiveness, placing it in the charge of the Universe or forces whose efficiency is unsuspected and unknown.

A remark by an interviewed person caught our attention, considering it an exercise in reflection on the essence of the human condition, placed in a situation that seems to be extreme - not so much through its dramatic dimensions, but especially through its novelty, which leaves room for imagination to create monsters or open doors to evolution, in the sense of awakening responsibility and awareness of everyone's place in society, as well as society's place in the ecosystem in which it exists. *I hope that we will give up a little of this arrogance specific to the species and understand that even if we are many, almost 8 billion, we are neither as strong, nor as intelligent, nor as well organized, nor as prepared as we like to believe.* (O.N.).

Cap. IV. Axial coding. The theoretical model generated regarding anguish and frustration experienced during the pandemic

Following the axial coding stage, the results obtained from the analysis of the interviews were recoded in the form of axial categories and thematic axes, which allows us to propose a theoretical model on the impact of the pandemic, from the perspective of anguish and anxiety experienced by a large part of the population.

IV.1. Analysis of results. Axial coding

The main axial categories we propose are:

• **Fear generated by the perceived risks of the pandemic** (high rate of morbidity and even mortality). The concept of risk society takes into account that, during this period, subjects are more aware than in previous epochs of the risks that appear in everyday life and to which they must adapt for good social functionality. The first risks highlighted were those related to one's own health and life.

• **Distrust in the authorities' ability to manage the pandemic and refusal of hospitalization**. Many respondents showed that they are afraid for their own health, which is why they refused hospitalization, even when they had suspicions - confirmed or not - of Covid-19 infection, because the Romanian healthcare system cannot cope with the pressure that the pandemic puts on this system.

• **Awareness of the accentuation of society's medicalization, awareness of current society as a "risk society".** The medicalized society represents that society in which each of us finds ourselves as potential patients.

• **Distrust in the real dimensions of the pandemic** and easier acceptance of fake news regarding the pandemic, against the background of the ambivalent attitude of the authorities.

• **Distrust in science** - especially in medical science - due to the appearance of contradictory news about possible treatments or therapeutic schemes, later invalidated. Another source of distrust in science is the partial non-compliance with ethical standards in research on human subjects, in order to create vaccines.

• **Distrust in public health systems and health authorities** - which is due to causes such as: lack of criteria for selecting patient prioritization, violations of patients' rights - through deprivation of treatment, involuntary hospitalization, violations of healthcare personnel rights (with direct reference to the situation of Suceava County Hospital); possible discrimination based on medical condition and health status, the risk of abuses related to medical practices (temperature measurement, wearing masks); the existence of the risk of authoritarian behaviors, interpreted as a "white dictatorship". All these violations are carried out in the name of the right to health and public good, without being, however, sufficiently explained in public communication.

• **General distrust in public authorities** - due to violations of rights such as freedom of movement - through closing borders, proposing a health passport, quarantine - including through measures insufficiently explained to the population; violations of religious freedom and conscience - including the prohibition of participation in Easter services and other religious ceremonies, public or private, weddings, baptisms, funerals.

• **Virtualization of social space** - transfer of educational, professional, medical activities online.

• **The constitutive elements of anguish generated by the pandemic** are: the character of social construction of specific forms of anguish, generated by the perception of risks of illness, loss of quality of life, diminishing social, personal and economic security, fear of the other - as a possible vector of infection -, distancing not only physical, but also social - in the sense of degradation of interpersonal communication and public trust, not only in the health system or public institutions, but also in each other.

• **Destructuring of sociability**; symbolic transfer of the mask, from a simple sanitary mask, to a social mask.

IV.2. Validation of research hypotheses and (bio)ethical reflections on the medicalization of social life

Within the ethical discourse, we have two main directions, initially a normative one (which is, in fact, a component of professional status, of the corpus of medical or professional knowledge in general), while another component refers to acceptability (ethical and, ultimately, social), to the way in which a medical phenomenon influences social life through the medicalization of society.

Therefore, the bioethical discourse should be outlined within a debate in the social sphere, but in which not only specialists from the medical field participate, but also from other branches - such as the sphere of public policies, health sociology and quality of life, philosophy, political science, and why not, law.

We note not only the role of bioethics in times of crisis, but also the profound crisis of bioethics, which in the current period has failed to maintain sociability, while society has failed to respect the principles of bioethics: ***the principle of beneficence, the principle of non-maleficence, respect for autonomy, social justice, respect for personal autonomy.***

Regarding the hypotheses / presuppositions from which the work started, following the analysis of the interviews, it was found that:

- ✓ In contradiction with the presupposition that the occurrence of states of anguish and anxiety during the pandemic period should be very frequent and that we should be able to detect various explicit symptoms of these states - possible anxiety disorders -, many responses were received in which subjects declare that they were not affected by the pandemic. Subsequently, however, some of them return and show that they actually lived distressing and stressful experiences during the pandemic period, but which they do not identify as such - in the form of sufferings or disorders -, as the subjects did not obviously manifest such symptoms of anxiety, which through externalization would be perceptible both for the subject and for those close to them, noting only changes in mental state or mood, which did not affect self-expression externally. This may express a resistance to frustration, which temporarily allows good coping, but which may generate long-term effects, in the form of possible phobias, resentments, etc.

- ✓ The main sources of anxiety highlighted were related to the interruption of daily activities, quarantine, the fact that people were forced to stay away from loved ones - which is, in our understanding, an extension of the idea of social distancing, from limiting physical proximity to limiting social communication.
- ✓ The hope of returning to normalcy represents, from our point of view, the attempt to humanize the pandemic experience. The humanization of the everyday is the key desideratum for post-pandemic society. Within this humanization of the everyday, a particularly important element is the elimination of fear from the foreground of relating to social life.

Responsibility towards others and towards one's own health condition is, in our opinion, a marker of the social construction of post-pandemic society as a risk society and of the accentuation of the medicalization of society, in the sense that the ***human condition itself will be perceived as a treatable disorder***, and the encounter with the Other will be perceived in the sense of encountering danger - in this case, with a possible source of infection.

A de-solidarized society generates an anguish of the presence of the other as a possible source of infection and which goes as far as to refuse its presence in the immediate vicinity, the subject itself being able to become the source of anguish, related to the depreciation of quality of life in correlation with the state of health.

IV.3. Medicalization of social life during pandemic

In the context of the COVID-19 pandemic, contemporary society has experienced an unprecedented intensification of the process of medicalization of social life. This phenomenon, characterized by the extension of medical authority over non-medical aspects of daily life, has taken on a particular magnitude, fundamentally transforming the way individuals and communities perceive and manage health, illness, and risk.

The process of medicalization, initially conceptualized by sociologists such as Irving Zola and Peter Conrad, refers to the tendency to define and treat most human problems as medical in nature. During the pandemic, this tendency has been dramatically accentuated, and the medical field has gained an overwhelming influence on political, economic, and social decisions. Public health measures, such as social distancing, mask-wearing, and quarantine, have radically reconfigured social interactions and placed medical considerations at the center of daily life.

The social construction of medicalization in the pandemic context has been influenced by multiple interconnected factors. Firstly, the uncertainty and fear generated by the new Coronavirus created fertile ground for the acceptance and even demand for extensive medical intervention in all spheres of life. Individuals, faced with an invisible and potentially lethal threat, sought refuge in medical expertise, conferring a central role to health authorities in crisis management.

Mass media played a crucial role in amplifying this process through the constant dissemination of medical information and pandemic-related statistics. News bulletins dominated by infection and death figures, along with dramatic images from hospitals, contributed to creating an atmosphere of permanent medical emergency. This informational saturation led to collective hypervigilance towards potential symptoms and risks, transforming each individual into a potential patient or disease transmission vector.

Public authorities adopted and promoted a predominantly medical discourse in crisis management, thus legitimizing the extension of social control based on medical reasons. Political and administrative decisions were justified by appealing to scientific and medical expertise, reinforcing the perception that solutions to complex social problems can be found in the medical field. This approach led to a redefinition of the concepts of normality and deviance in medical terms, with compliant behaviors being equated with responsibility towards public health.

In the economic sphere, medicalization manifested through the reconfiguration of business priorities and practices around public health imperatives. Companies had to adapt their operations to comply with health protocols, and economic sectors were classified and regulated according to their degree of "essentiality" from a public health perspective. This realignment of economic priorities with medical ones reinforced the perception that health, in a broad sense, is the foundation of society's functioning.

In the field of education, the transition to online learning brought medical considerations to the forefront in organizing the educational process. Decisions regarding school openings or closures, implementation of protective measures, and curriculum adaptation were predominantly guided by medical reasons, underlining the extension of medical authority into the educational sphere.

At the individual level, medicalization manifested through intensified self-monitoring and health concern. Individuals adopted rigorous hygiene practices, constantly monitored potential symptoms, and internalized a medical discourse in evaluating their own behaviors and those of others. This medical hypervigilance led to a redefinition of personal and social identity in terms of medical risk and health responsibility.

The social construction of medicalization in the pandemic was also facilitated by technological advances in the medical and communications fields. The rapid development of vaccines and diagnostic tests, along with the widespread implementation of contact tracing applications, reinforced confidence in medical and technological solutions for social problems. This convergence between medicine, technology, and social control amplified the perception that social life can and should be managed through medical instruments.

The phenomenon of medicalization in the pandemic also generated a series of social tensions and contradictions. On one hand, it led to an unprecedented mobilization of resources and solidarity around public health objectives. On the other hand, it exacerbated existing inequalities and created new forms of marginalization and stigmatization based on medical criteria. Vulnerable groups, already disadvantaged, faced additional barriers in accessing resources and opportunities, justified by public health reasons.

Moreover, the intense medicalization of social life generated reactions of resistance and contestation. Anti-vaccine movements and protests against restrictive measures represented forms of opposition to extended medical authority and the redefinition of individual freedoms in medical terms. These tensions highlighted the limits and potential dangers of an exclusively medicalized approach to complex social problems.

The social construction of medicalization in the pandemic context was also influenced by specific cultural and historical factors. In societies with a strong tradition of individualism and personal freedom, the process of medicalization encountered more resistance, being perceived as a form of excessive social control. In contrast, in cultures with a more collectivist orientation or with historical experiences of managing public health crises, medicalization was more easily accepted and internalized.

An important aspect of the social construction of medicalization in the pandemic was the reconfiguration of public and private space through the lens of medical considerations. Social distancing and mobility restrictions dramatically transformed the urban landscape and social practices, introducing new norms of interaction based on health imperatives. Public spaces were reorganized to facilitate physical distancing, and the boundary between public and private space became more fluid, with homes often transforming into workplaces, schools, and virtual medical centers.

The public discourse dominated by medical expertise led to a redefinition of risk and security concepts in predominantly medical terms. National and individual security was reinterpreted through the lens of threats to public health, justifying unprecedented surveillance and control measures in peacetime. This fusion between medical and security discourse amplified the perception of a permanent state of emergency, legitimizing the extension of medical authority into spheres traditionally separate from medicine.

In the sphere of interpersonal relationships, medicalization manifested through the introduction of new rituals and norms of interaction based on medical considerations. Traditional greetings were replaced with "safe" gestures from a health perspective, and expressions of affection and intimacy were redefined in the context of virus transmission risk. These changes had a profound impact on how individuals construct and maintain social relationships, introducing a medical dimension into the most intimate aspects of daily life.

The process of medicalization has also influenced the perception of time and the future. Uncertainty related to the pandemic's evolution has led to an intense focus on the present and immediate management of medical risks, to the detriment of long-term planning. The future began to be conceptualized predominantly in terms of epidemiological scenarios, and personal and social plans were subordinated to public health considerations.

In the professional sphere, medicalization manifested through redefining the concept of work and work relationships through the lens of medical risk. Telework became the norm in many sectors, and workplace safety acquired a strong medical dimension. This reconfiguration led to the emergence of new forms of inequality and vulnerability based on the possibility or impossibility of working remotely and the degree of exposure to medical risks in professional activity.

The social construction of medicalization in the pandemic was also amplified by the phenomenon of "infodemic" - the rapid proliferation of information, both correct and false, about the virus and pandemic. This constant flow of medical information contributed to maintaining a state of permanent alert and consolidating the authority of medical discourse in interpreting social reality. At the same time, it generated confusion and anxiety, fueling conspiracy theories and challenging scientific authority.

An important aspect of medicalization in the pandemic context was the extension of the concept of individual responsibility in the field of public health. Individuals were called to assume an active role in preventing the spread of the virus, transforming each daily decision into a potential public health intervention. This individual responsibilization reinforced the perception that health is a matter of personal choice and responsible behavior, partially obscuring the social and structural factors that influence population health.

In conclusion, the social construction of medicalization of social life in the context of the COVID-19 pandemic represents a complex phenomenon that has fundamentally transformed the way society conceptualizes and manages health, risk, and social relationships. This process has led to an unprecedented extension of medical authority in all spheres of life, redefining fundamental concepts such as normality, freedom, and social responsibility through the lens of health imperatives.

The long-term implications of this intensification of medicalization remain to be fully understood and evaluated. On one hand, it has led to an impressive mobilization of resources and solidarity in the face of a global threat, demonstrating society's capacity to adapt rapidly in the face of crises. On the other hand, it has raised important questions about the balance between public health and other fundamental social values, such as individual freedom and equity.

In the post-pandemic period, society faces the challenge of negotiating a new balance between medical imperatives and other social priorities. This process requires critical reflection on the limits and consequences of extensive medicalization of social life, as well as a re-evaluation of how we conceptualize health and illness in a social context. A deep understanding of how the phenomenon of medicalization was socially constructed during the pandemic will be essential for overcoming these challenges and building more balanced and inclusive approaches to public health in the future.

Cap V. Philosophical counseling in the context of the accentuated medicalization of society

The medicalization of society essentially represents an effect of the "risk society," reflecting an accentuated awareness of various threats perceived by individuals. This phenomenon leads to the conceptualization of the human condition as a "treatable disorder," illustrating the extension of the medical paradigm over fundamental aspects of existence.

V.1. Medicalization of society and its impact on the social life

In the context of the pandemic, we have witnessed an unprecedented restriction of social activity, with emphasis on social distancing - a term that the World Health Organization proposes to replace with physical distancing, recognizing the importance of maintaining social communication.

The accelerated virtualization of social interactions, although necessary to combat the spread of COVID-19, had the potential to generate real social distancing, concurrent with physical distancing. This phenomenon manifested through an interpretative drift of the risk society construct into one of a deeply medicalized society, where public health imperatives prevail over economic and social development considerations. Without criticizing this prioritization, we must recognize that the medicalization of social life promotes a lifestyle centered on sometimes exaggerated concern for health status, manifested through increased consumption of pharmaceutical products or natural alternatives presumed to have miraculous effects.

The proliferation of so-called healthy and organic lifestyles reflects collective anxiety related to the potential loss of comfort and health, in the context of increased awareness of daily risks. Many of these efforts, however, prove superficial, generating the illusion of a healthy life. In this context, ethical and philosophical counseling can offer a different perspective on the real impact of these risks on our lives, reducing both the consumption of self-administered medicinal products and the existential anguish that appears in the context of the risk society. We align here with Lou Marinoff's opinion formulated in the volume "Plato, Not Prozac!" (Marinoff, 2019) which suggests a counseling solution consisting of philosophical practice to replace self-medication and eliminate excessive medicalization of social life.

Responding to concerns about the crisis of philosophy, manifested through reduced public adherence to traditional domains of the discipline, philosopher Lou Marinoff attributes this situation to the ossification of traditional academic discourse, the elitist approach to philosophy, and the relative incompatibility of fundamental themes of contemporary philosophy with the everyday intellectual concerns of potential readers.

V.2. Philosophical practice as alternative to excessive medicalization

Philosophical practice emerges as a potential solution to the crisis of academic philosophy, proposing an innovative approach to philosophy that aims to return to the love of wisdom and reposition philosophy in the agora, far from the ivory tower of academic approach. The anti-academic and anti-epistemic character of philosophical practice is accentuated by criticisms of traditional academic philosophy by thinkers such as Achenbach and Hadot, who emphasize the deviation of philosophy's meaning towards a discourse limited to classical themes, often sterile and inadequate for society's current concerns. On the other hand, we cannot fail to notice the profoundly intellectual character of many so-called pragmatic discourses, which emphasize concerns for the everyday, including those we understand under the term medicalization of social life, and which make it difficult for the individual to detach from the immediate, the contextual, and the contingent.

Philosophical counseling, a form of philosophical practice, presents itself as a therapy of the spirit that uses the resources of practical wisdom for an alternative approach to the human condition, thus contrasting with the medicalization of social life. Lou Marinoff, in the aforementioned work, argues that philosophical practice represents a way out of the medicalization of society, suggesting that many forms of depression and anxiety, except for those deeply based on significant chemical imbalances, could be more effectively addressed through philosophical reflection and conscious living, rather than through psychotropic medication.

This perspective does not imply abandoning medical advice, but rather a re-evaluation of excessive dependence on medical and especially pseudo-scientific interventions, which abound in contemporary society and are often products of aggressive marketing from the pharmaceutical industry. It is important to emphasize that this approach should not be confused with the refusal of any medication or with the acceptance of conspiracy theories that place the pharmaceutical industry at the origin of significant epidemics (Sandu, 2019).

The effort to confront oneself and existential anxiety is essential for achieving authentic satisfaction in life. Paradoxical happiness, supported more by external medical efforts than by personal reflection and inner dialogue, can lead to persistent dissatisfaction. The medicalization of social life, in this context, represents an excessive use of instruments originating from the medical sphere, inadequately adapted to everyday life, which profoundly mark our daily existence.

Philosophical practice is proposed as an alternative to the excessive medicalization of social life, offering a framework for exploring and addressing existential problems through philosophical reflection and dialogue, both with oneself and with others.

V.3. "Healthy" lifestyles and medicalization in the eco-ethical context

Yoga practice represents an eloquent example of the tendencies towards medicalization of social life. Initially conceived as an ascetic practice dedicated to self-knowledge and union with the Divine, contemporary yoga has frequently been reduced to a form of gymnastics meant to offer mental comfort and an illusion of health effort. The transformation of yoga from a profound spiritual discipline into a superficial physical activity illustrates the deviation from its original purpose and its integration into the healthy lifestyle industry.

The organic and bio-food phenomenon also reflects this tendency towards medicalization. Although the consumption of naturally produced foods presents undeniable benefits, the organic industry has often become a pretext for marketing products at exorbitant prices, without a real guarantee of quality or natural production methods. This situation raises significant ethical and ecological questions regarding the authenticity and real impact of these practices on health and the environment.

From an eco-ethical perspective, we need a critical reflection on the effective lifestyle changes generated by the purchase of expensive organic products, in the absence of broader measures to reduce pollution and improve quality of life. Instead of adopting coherent public policies that reflect an ethic of relationships with nature, individual measures are promoted for adopting a naturist or organic lifestyle, which, in reality, contribute to creating a new industry that exploits the fear of illness.

The fitness industries, sometimes renamed as "yoga," and the organic and bio-product industry largely produce pseudo-natural artifacts, speculating on the socially internalized fear of disease. This fear is a social construct based on the perception that our life depends on environmental conditions that we cannot fully control, except by returning to nature, a nature that is, however, partially degraded by human activity.

In the context of this tendency towards medicalization of social life, where genuine concern for health and environment is often replaced with commercial practices that exploit collective anxieties, without really addressing fundamental issues of public health and ecology. An ethical approach would require a profound awareness of the ecological situation and the implementation of comprehensive measures at a societal level, instead of the superficial individual solutions currently promoted.

In contemporary society, we have become accustomed to a certain level of comfort and a minimization of discomfort, which has led to an accentuation of the fear of illness and suffering, in contrast with previous generations. This paradigm shift is based on a profound transformation in the perception and management of health risks, illustrating the tendency we define through the term medicalization of social life.

Unlike previous historical periods, when confrontation with mortality and suffering was a daily reality, current society manifests an increased dependence on medical intervention for any minor discomfort. This attitude, although beneficial in many respects, represents a symptom of excessive medicalization of social life, where social decisions are predominantly guided by medical considerations, sometimes to the detriment of other important social aspects.

Lou Marinoff argues against the passive acceptance of this dependence on the medical system, advocating for a philosophical approach, especially regarding mental health and social life. He suggests limiting, although not completely eliminating, the medical approach that tends to see the individual more as a patient than as a person integrated into a complex of psycho-social interactions.

We distinguish between real mental disorders and existential anxiety. The tendency to medicalize every aspect of psychic life, from psychoses to everyday neurotic manifestations, risks leading to a pharmacological suppression of states of emotional discomfort, with the potential to erode the fundamental capacity for self-reflection and self-knowledge.

The critique of excessive medicalization does not imply a rejection of evidence-based medical practice, but rather a plea for reducing therapeutic excess and the tendency to interpret any social and communicational phenomenon through the lens of pathology. Instead, an approach is proposed that integrates the philosophical, self-reflective perspective in managing anxieties and depressions with existential origins, as is the case with those generated by pandemic phenomena.

We suggest that a lifestyle based on self-knowledge and self-analysis can represent an essential component of quality of life, offering an alternative, a valuable complement to the strictly medical approach to psychological discomfort. This perspective invites a re-evaluation of how society conceptualizes and approaches mental health, suggesting an integration of medical considerations with philosophical and existential ones in managing individual and collective well-being.

V.4. Philosophical and ethical counseling in post-pandemic society

Philosophical counseling thus emerges as a viable alternative to the excessive medicalization of social life, without diminishing the real importance of medical intervention in justified cases. This approach emphasizes psychotherapeutic treatment and philosophical reflection, especially in situations where an individual's anxieties do not have a biological basis but are generated by existential dilemmas or the inability to cope with life's challenges.

Unlike the traditional psychotherapeutic approach, we appreciate that philosophical practice abandons the deficiency paradigm specific to the medical model, replacing it with that of existential dilemmas. This practice aims to stimulate the individual's reflection on their own life and personal value system, transforming the client from a presumed patient into a seeker of practical wisdom.

The Socratic dialogue method and maieutics are central tools of philosophical counseling, facilitating a deep exploration of personal philosophical consciousness and the assumed meaning of existence. This approach proves particularly useful in growth crisis situations, when the individual must relate to transcendence and their own position in the universe.

In the current context, marked by an increased dependence on medical resources, philosophical counseling proposes a way to interrogatively relate to the meanings we attribute to life, to discover our own presuppositions, and to develop critical thinking. It offers an alternative to the loss of the ability to relate to the finitude of existence in a heroic manner, characteristic of previous epochs.

The exceptional situation generated by the global pandemic brings to the forefront the model of the savior hero, exemplified by medical personnel on the front lines of the fight against COVID-19. These manifestations of everyday heroism compel us to reposition ourselves and rethink the personal and collective myths that motivate and justify our existence.

We propose that philosophical practice adopt a narrative and appreciative approach, analyzing the stories we tell ourselves to justify our existence and how we incorporate fundamental myths that generate behaviors and ways of thinking. The aggregation of individual narratives into constitutive metanarratives of society, based on ethical values, becomes essential.

The re-emergence of heroism as a constitutive value at the societal level underlines the need to reawaken in ourselves the capacity to give, to communicate, and to empathize with others. Philosophical counseling, through its reflective and critical approach, offers a propitious framework for exploring and integrating these values into everyday life, thus contributing to a deeper understanding of the human condition in the context of contemporary challenges, including pandemic ones but not limited to these.

Humanity faces, especially following the pandemic experience, an acute reminder of courage as a constitutive ethical value of modern society, a value that, until recently, was perceived predominantly through the lens of chivalric myths or Hollywood narratives. This value suddenly becomes fundamental for post-pandemic society, operationalizing itself through stories of everyday heroes.

Beyond these constitutive values of post- and trans-modern society, the necessity of its operational values - such as prudence - emerges to guide the practical implementation of courage. In the medical field, for example, courage must be doubled by wisdom and prudence, ensuring that frontline medical personnel, during the pandemic period for instance, benefit from necessary protective equipment.

Philosophical and ethical counseling should emphasize these values and identify moments from the subject's previous experience where they experienced courage and prudence as constitutive values of the social or professional practices in which they are involved. These values, although highlighted in medical practice in the current period, are relevant in other areas of daily life as well, such as social assistance or public administration.

The interference between bioethics and philosophical counseling materializes in the concept of ethical counseling, which encompasses, besides proper ethical values, certain spiritual values. These values can be explored from the perspective of the philosopher-counselor who understands the relationship with the Divine as a possible relation to alterity, within the limits of awareness of our own finitude and our position in the world.

This holistic approach, which combines philosophical reflection with ethical and spiritual considerations, provides a referential framework for facing the complex challenges of contemporary society, especially in the context of global crises such as the pandemic. It allows for a re-evaluation of fundamental values and a recalibration of how we relate to our own existence and our relationship with others and the surrounding world.

Conclusions

Among the most important results obtained from the analysis of the interviews, we enumerate: the awareness of the accentuation of society's medicalization, the awareness of current society as a "risk society," distrust in the authorities' ability to manage the pandemic, distrust in the real dimensions of the pandemic and easier acceptance of fake news regarding the pandemic, against the background of the ambivalent attitude of authorities, refusal of hospitalization - even in the context of Covid-19 infection - justified by the perception of the Romanian medical system's inability to manage the crisis, as well as the existence of the risk of authoritarian behaviors, interpreted as a "white dictatorship."

The medicalization of society represents an effect of the perception of postmodern society as a risk society. In the risk society, community members more easily become aware of the various types of risks by which individuals feel threatened. When the medicalization of society becomes a mass phenomenon, it can lead to the idea of medicalization of the human condition, with individuals' humanity being considered a treatable syndrome.

The general conclusion of this research was that we have moved towards another period, based on what we call the virtualization of social space and interactions, and this virtualization affects family life.

Life in a medicalized society can at a certain point be a flight from any risks, but once it reaches paroxysm, it can eliminate the subjective quality of life, for the sake of a so-called objective quality, measured in an apparent state of health, translated by the absence of an acute infection, but with the permanent presence of social or psychological dysfunctions.

Acknowledgement

Parts of the research underlying this volume have been partially published previously in scientific articles, as follows:

Sandu, A. (2020). The Medicalization of the Social Life, 34-51, *Revista de Filosofie Aplicată*, [S.l.], v. 3, june 2020. ISSN 2668-0009. Disponibil la:https://filosofieaplicata.ro/index.php/filap/article/view/47/37

Sandu, A. (2021). Anxiety and Frustration During the Covid-19 Pandemic. *Archiv Euromedica* 11(6), pp. 10-15. http://dx.doi.org/10.35630/2199-885X/2021/11/6.2

Sandu, A. (2018). *Abordări calitative în cercetarea socială. Teoria fundamentată pe date (Grounded Theory)* [Qualitative approaches in social research. Grounded Theory]. Lumen, Romania

Sandu, A. (2020). Pandemic - Catalyst of the Virtualization of the Social Space, *Postmodern Openings*, Editura Lumen, Department of Economics, vol. 11(1Sup2), pages 115-140. https://doi.org/10.18662/po/11.1sup2/146

Sandu, A. (2021). Identity Changes in Crisis Situations. Anxiety, Frustration and Anguish Due to The Covid-19 Pandemic. *Analele Ştiinţifice ale Universităţii »Alexandru Ioan Cuza« din Iaşi. Sociologie şi Asistenţă Socială*, 14/2021 (2), pp.17-28

Sandu, A. (2023). Social Construction of a Pandemic. Medicalization of Social Life - Anxiety, Frustration and Ethical Risks BRAIN. *Broad Research in Artificial Intelligence and Neuroscience,* 14(2), 165-197. https://doi.org/10.18662/brain/14.2/450

References

Academia Română, Institutul de Lingvistică. (2009). *Dicţionarul explicativ al limbii române* (2nd ed.). Editura Univers Enciclopedic Gold [Romanian Academy, Institute of Linguistics (2009). Explanatory dictionary of Romanian language] . https://dexonline.ro/definitie/anxietate

Adam, S. (2009). Profesia de cadru didactic între reprezentare socială şi vocaţie individuală [Teaching profession between social representation and individual vocation]. *Revista de Cercetare în Ştiinţe ale Educaţiei.* http://www.rcsedu.info/index.php?option=com_content&view=article&id=17:profesia-de-cadru-didactic-intre-reprezentare-social-i-vocaie-individual&catid=10:sociologia-educaiei-

American Psychiatric Association (APA). (2013). *The Diagnostic and Statistical Manual of Mental Disorders* (5th ed.) (DSM5). Washington, DC.

Bao, Y., Sun, Y., Meng, S., Shi, J., & Lu, L. (2020). 2019-nCoV Epidemic: Address Mental Health Care to Empower Society. *The Lancet*, 395(10224), e37–e38. https://doi.org/10.1016/S0140-6736(20)30309-3

Basheti, I. A., Mhaidat, Q. N., & Mhaidat, H. N. (2021). Prevalence of Anxiety and Depression During COVID-19 Pandemic Among Healthcare Students in Jordan and Its Effect on Their

Learning Process: A National Survey. *PLoS ONE*, 16(4), e0249716. https://doi.org/10.1371/journal.pone.0249716

Beck, A. (1976). *Cognitive therapy and the emotional disorders*. International Universities Press.

Beck, U. (1992). *Risk Society: Towards a New Modernity*. Sage.

Boccaccio, G. (2003). *The Decameron* (2nd ed.). Penguin Books.

Bowlby, J. (1969). *Attachment and loss: Vol. 1. Attachment*. Basic Books.

Bronfenbrenner, U. (1979). *The ecology of human development*. Harvard University Press.

Brooks, S. K., Webster, R. K., Smith, L. E., Woodland, L., Wessely, S., Greenberg, N., & Rubin, G. J. (2020). The Psychological Impact of Quarantine and How to Reduce It: Rapid Review of the Evidence. *The Lancet*, 395(10227), 912–920. https://doi.org/10.1016/S0140-6736(20)30460-8

Bystritsky, A., Khalsa, S. S., Cameron, M. E., & Schiffman, J. (2013). Current Diagnosis and Treatment of Anxiety Disorders. *P & T : A Peer-Reviewed Journal For Formulary Management*, 38(1), 30–57.

Conrad, P. (2007). *The Medicalization of Society: On the transformation of Human Conditions into Treatable Disorders*. The John Hopkins University Press.

Corbin, J., & Strauss, A. (2008). *Basics of Qualitative Research: Techniques and Procedures for Developing Grounded Theory* (3rd ed.). Sage Publications.

Creswell, J. W. (2007). *Qualitative Inquiry and Research Design: Choosing Among Five Traditions* (2nd ed.). Sage Publications.

Delumeau, J. (2021). *Frica în Occident. Secolele XIV - XVIII. O cetate asediată* [Fear in the West. 14th - 18th Centuries. A Besieged Fortress]. Art.

Dorofte, T. (1991). *Orientari si tendinte in psihoterapia contemporana* [Orientations and trends in contemporary psychotherapy]. Editura Stiintifica, Romania

Dorofte, T. (1997). *Dimensiuni socio-psihologice ale personalitatii* [Socio-psychological dimensions of personality]. Pro Humanitate, Romania

Ekberg, M. (2007). The Parameters of the Risk Society: A Review and Exploration. *Current Sociology*, 55(3), 343–366. https://doi.org/10.1177/0011392107076080

Ellis, A. (1995). Changing rational-emotive therapy (RET) to rational emotive behavior therapy (REBT). *Journal of Rational-Emotive & Cognitive-Behavior Therapy*, 13(2), 85-89. https://doi.org/10.1007/BF02354453

Foucault, M. (2010). *The Birth of Biopolitics: Lectures at the Collège de France, 1978--1979 (Lectures at the College de France)*. Picador.

Freud, S. (2010). *Psihopatologia vieţii cotidiene. Despre uitare, greşeli de vorbire, superstiţie şi eroare* [The Psychopathology of Everyday Life. On Forgetfulness, Mispronunciation, Superstition, and Error]. Trei, Romania

Goulding, C. (1999). *Grounded Theory: Some Reflections on Paradigm, Procedures and Misconceptions*. Working Paper Series, Wolverhampton Business School, Management Research Centre. http://hdl.handle.net/2436/11403

Hall, R. C. W., Hall, R. C. W., & Chapman, M. J. (2008). The 1995 Kikwit Ebola Outbreak: Lessons Hospitals and Physicians Can Apply to Future Viral Epidemics. *General Hospital Psychiatry*, 30(5), 446–452. https://doi.org/10.1016/j.genhosppsych.2008.05.003

Heimberg, R. G., Hofmann, S. G., Liebowitz, M. R., Schneier, F. R., Smits, J. A. J., Stein, M. B., Hinton, D. E., & Craske, M. G. (2014). Social Anxiety Disorder in DSM-5. *Depression and Anxiety*, 31(6), 472-479. https://doi.org/10.1002/da.22231

Kessler, R. C., McGonagle, K. A., Zhao, S., Nelson, C. B., Hughes, M., Eshleman, S., Wittchen, H. U., & Kendler, K. S. (1994). Lifetime and 12-Month Prevalence of DSM-III-R Psychiatric Disorders in the United States. Results From the National Comorbidity Survey. *Arch Gen Psychiatry*, 51(1), 8-19. https://doi.org/10.1001/archpsyc.1994.03950010008002

Korkmaz, H., & Güloğlu, B. (2021). The Role of Uncertainty Tolerance and Meaning in Life on Depression and Anxiety Throughout Covid-19 Pandemic. *Personality and Individual Differences*, 179, 110952. https://doi.org/10.1016/j.paid.2021.110952

Kristoffersen, E. S., Faiz, K. W., Sandset, E. C., Storstein, A. M., Stefansen, S., Winsvold, B. S., & Hansen, J. M. (2020). Hospital-Based Headache Care During the Covid-19 Pandemic in Denmark and Norway. *The Journal of Headache and Pain*, 21(1), 128. http://dx.doi.org/10.1186/s10194-020-01195-2

Lazarus, R., & Folkman, S. (1984). *Stress, appraisal and coping*. Springer.

Leon, A. C., Portera, L., & Weissman, M. M. (1995). The Social Costs of Anxiety Disorders. *The British Journal of Psychiatry*, 166(27), 19-22. https://doi.org/10.1192/S0007125000293355

Marinoff, L. (2019). *Înghite Platon, nu prozac!* [Plato, not Prozac!] Trei, Romania

Medicover. (n.d.). *Cele mai frecvente tulburări anxioase și cum le gestionăm* [The most common anxiety disorders and how to manage them]. https://www.medicover.ro/despre-sanatate/cele-mai-frecvente-tulburari-anxioase-si-cum-le-gestionam,145,n,292

Miftofe, V. (2010). *Tratat de asistenta sociala. Protectia populatiilor specifice si automarginalizate* [Social assistance treaty.

Protection of specific and self-marginalized populations]. Lumen, Romania

NODEX - Noul dicţionar explicativ al limbii române [The new explanatory dictionary of Romanian language]. (2002). Editura Litera Internaţional, Romania https://dexonline.ro/definitie/anxietate

Ozamiz-Etxebarria, N., Dosil-Santamaria, M., Picaza-Gorrochategui, M., & Idoiaga-Mondragon, N. (2020). Stress, Anxiety, and Depression Levels in the Initial Stage of the COVID-19 Outbreak in a Population Sample in the Northern Spain. *Cad Saude Publica*, *36*(4), e00054020. https://doi.org/10.1590/0102-311X00054020

Porter, D. (n.d.). Social Anxiety Disorder (Social Phobia), *DSM-5* 300.23 (F40.10). https://www.theravive.com/therapedia/social-anxiety-disorder-(social-phobia)-dsm--5-300.-23-(f40.10)?fbclid=IwAR3RIOIl6Lt4xiXCQ-X3eBwcJS-sMiJoaSr2IggXM8fJGbRLr08C9-GERtMMY

Reynolds, C. R., & Kamphaus, R. W. (2013). *Generalized Anxiety Disorder*. American Psychiatric Association.

Rizzoli, P. B., & Grazzi, L. (2020). The Adaptation of Management of Chronic Migraine Patients With Medication Overuse to the Suspension of Treatment Protocols During the COVID-19 Pandemic: Lessons From a Tertiary Headache Center in Milan, Italy. *Headache, 60*(7), 1463–1464. https://doi.org/10.1111/head.14140

Salari, N., Hosseinian-Far, A., Jalali, R., Vaisi-Raygani, A., Rasoulpoor, S., Mohammadi, M., Rasoulpoor, S., & Khaledi-Paveh, B. (2020). Prevalence of Stress, Anxiety, Depression Among the General Population During the COVID-19 Pandemic: A Systematic Review and Meta-Analysis. *Globalization and Health, 16*(57). https://doi.org/10.1186/s12992-020-00589-w

Sandu, A. (2010). Freedom as a Hermeneutical Pretext. *Revista Românească pentru Educație Multidimensională, 2*(3), 5-24. https://revistaromaneasca.ro/freedom-as-a-hermeneutical-pretext/

Sandu, A. (2018). *Abordări calitative în cercetarea socială. Teoria fundamentată pe date (Grounded Theory)* [Qualitative approaches in social research. Grounded Theory]. Lumen, Romania

Sandu, A. (2019). *Consilierea filosofică apreciativă* [Appreciative philosophical counseling]. Lumen, Romania

Sandu, A. (2020). *Bioetica în criză sau criza bioeticii? O filosofie a societății medicalizate* [Bioethics in crisis or the crisis of bioethics? A philosophy of the medicalized society]. Lumen, Romania

Sandu, A. (2020). The Medicalization of the Social Life. *Revista de Filosofie Aplicată*, 3, 34-51. https://filosofieaplicata.ro/index.php/filap/article/view/47/37

Sandu, A. (2020). Pandemic - Catalyst of the Virtualization of the Social Space, *Postmodern Openings*, 11(1Sup2)/2020, 115-140. https://doi.org/10.18662/po/11.1sup2/146

Sandu, A. (2021). Anxiety and Frustration During the Covid-19 Pandemic. *Archiv Euromedica*, 11(6), 10-15. http://dx.doi.org/10.35630/2199-885X/2021/11/6.2

Sandu, A. (2021). Identity Changes in Crisis Situations. Anxiety, Frustration and Anguish Due to The Covid-19 Pandemic. *Analele Ştiinţifice ale Universităţii »Alexandru Ioan Cuza« din Iaşi. Sociologie şi Asistenţă Socială*, 14/2021 (2), 17-28

Sandu, A. (2023). Social Construction of a Pandemic. Medicalization of Social Life - Anxiety, Frustration and Ethical Risks BRAIN. *Broad Research in Artificial Intelligence and Neuroscience,* 14(2), 165-197. https://doi.org/10.18662/brain/14.2/450

Shigemura, J., Ursano, R. J., Morganstein, J. C., Kurosawa, M., & Benedek, D. M. (2020). Public Responses to the Novel 2019 Coronavirus (2019-NCOV) in Japan: Mental Health Consequences and Target Populations. *Psychiatry and Clinical Neurosciences*, 74(4), 281. https://doi.org/10.1111/pcn.12988

Suzuki, K., Takeshima, T., Igarashi, H., Imai, N., Danno, D., Yamamoto, T., Nagata, E., Haruyama, Y., Mitsufuji, T., Suzuki, S., Ito, Y., Shibata, M., Kowa, H., Kikui, S., Shiina,

T., Okamura, M., Tatsumoto, M., & Hirata, K. (2021). Impact of the COVID-19 Pandemic on Migraine in Japan: A Multicentre Crosssectional Study. The *Journal of Headache and Pain*, 22(53). https://doi.org/10.1186/s10194-021-012-63-1

Tedeschi, R., & Calhoun, L. (2004). Posttraumatic growth: conceptual foundations and empirical evidence. *Psychological Inquiry*, 15(1), 1-18. https://doi.org/10.1207/s15327965pli1501_01

Williams, S. J., & Calnan, M. (1996). The 'Limits' of Medicalization?: Modern Medicine and the Lay Populace In 'Late' Modernity. *Social Science and Medicine*, 42(12), 1609-1620. https://doi.org/10.1016/0277-9536(95)00313-4

World Health Organization (WHO) (2001). *Strengthening mental health promotion,* Fact sheet No 220. http://www.who.int/mediacentre/factsheets/fs220/en/

Xiang, Y. T., Yang, Y., Li, W., Zhang, L., Zhang, Q., Cheung, T., & Ng, C. H. (2020). Timely Mental Health Care For the 2019 Novel Coronavirus Outbreak Is Urgently Needed. *Lancet Psychiatry, 7*(3), 228–229.

Zhang, J., Lu, H., Zeng, H., Zhang, S., Du, Q., Jiang, T., & Dua, B. (2020). The Differential Psychological Distress of Populations Affected By the COVID-19 Pandemic. *Brain, Behavior, and Immunity*, 87, 49–50. https://doi.org/10.1016/j.bbi.2020.04.031

Anexes

Interview Guide #1

Interview guide applied to Romanian citizens in the diaspora who were outside Romania's territory during the pandemic period.

1. What is your age?
2. What is your level of education?
3. In which country are you/were you during the pandemic?
4. What is your opinion about the Coronavirus pandemic?
5. What were the main measures adopted by the authorities of the country where you were/are?
6. What is your opinion regarding these measures, are they necessary or not?
7. To what extent did you respect these measures? Do you intend to respect them from now on?
8. Please detail your emotional state that persisted/ persists during this period.
9. What were your biggest fears regarding the medical system in the country where you were/are?
10. To what extent has this pandemic affected your financial situation?
11. How have social distancing measures affected you?
12. If you are among Romanians in the diaspora, what were your main concerns when you learned about the spread of this pandemic?

Interview Guide #2

Interview guide applied to people who were infected with Covid-19 during the pandemic period or suffered from comorbidities that placed them in a vulnerable category of the population:

1. Can you please tell me your age?
2. Do you suffer from any particular illness?
3. Please describe a typical day in your life.
4. In terms of home isolation, how did you manage to adapt to this situation?
5. During this period, did you experience feelings of fear/anxiety and/or concern regarding your health and that of your loved ones? If yes, how did you manage to control it?
6. Do you usually talk about the feelings or thoughts you are facing during this period?
7. Can you tell me about the most difficult period you faced during isolation?
8. We all want at some point to have a period of quiet, staying at home, however when this is forced by circumstances, it can become a burden. How do you think we can ease this task during this period? (activity recommendations)
9. During this period, did you feel useless, that you are no longer able to do certain things you used to do before, or simply revolt against the situation you were in? If yes, how did you overcome these feelings?
10. Do you have any uncertainty about what the future holds for you? If yes, how do you think things you were used to before the pandemic will change?

11. From an economic and professional point of view, how do you feel during this period?
12. We have been talking about the negative aspects you experienced during this period due to isolation, however, do you think this virus has also brought benefits?

Interview Guide #3

Interview guide applied to people who faced financial problems, job loss, temporary unemployment, etc.

1. Please tell me how you view the measures imposed by Military Ordinance no. 3/24.03.2020
2. What is your opinion about this virus?
3. How are you isolating yourself with your family?
4. How will you cope with this emergency period, given that the movement of people is limited?
5. How will elderly people endure?
6. What is your opinion about the sanctions imposed by this Military Ordinance?
7. What do you think about the filing of criminal cases for those who do not respect the isolation/ quarantine measure?

Interview Guide #4

Interview guide applied to people who are caring for elderly, sick persons, or other family members:

1. Please specify your age.
2. What is your level of education?
3. Please specify your background environment.
4. What precautionary measures are you applying during this period?
5. How do you feel about not being able to carry out your activities as usual, due to the restrictions?
6. How have your planned projects been influenced during this period of isolation?
7. What is your mental state following the effects caused by the coronavirus?
8. Do you think there will be major changes following this pandemic? Will everything return to normal?

About the author

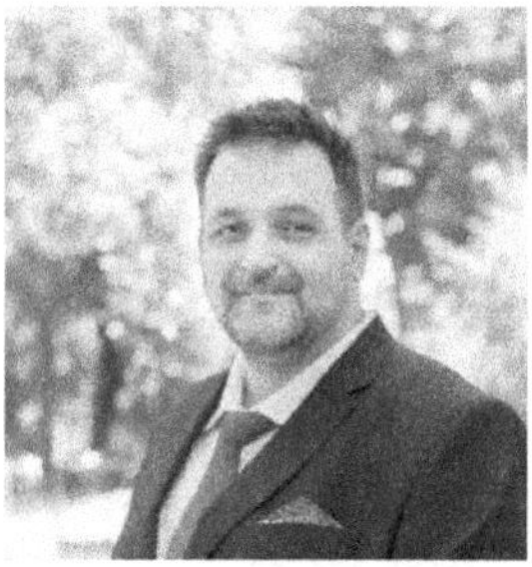

Antonio SANDU is a full professor at "Stefan cel Mare" University of Suceava, Romania, a senior researcher at the LUMEN Research Center in Social and Humanistic Sciences, Iasi, Romania, a professor and doctoral coordinator at the University of Oradea, and also the director of LUMEN Publishing House, Iasi, Romania. His main areas of interest include ethics, bioethics, sociology, social work, and social philosophy, public administration. The original contributions of the author's scientific activities stem from the social construction of reality seen from a semiological perspective. He analyzes the social construction of reality by developing his own version of this paradigm that operates at the intersection between it and the theory of communicative action. He has studied the interpretative drift of ethical concepts such as ethical acceptability and ethical values. He has conducted research on autonomy and informed consent in the field of medical ethics and public health ethics. He is also interested in the changes undergone by the human condition under the influence of the virtualization of social space and humanity's transition to a trans and posthuman stage. He is the author of the volume Bioethics in Crisis or the Crisis of Bioethics? An Anthropology of the

Pandemic in the Medicalized Society, published by Lumen Publishing House. He has also published the volume Social Construction of Reality as Communicative Action, published by Cambridge Scholar Publishing (2016), as well as the volumes Social Work Practice: Research Techniques and Intervention Models, Appreciative Ethics: A Constructionist Version of Ethics and Social-Constructionist Epistemology: A Transmodern Overview. The last three books were published by Lap Lambert between 2012 - 2013. He is the coordinator of the books Ethical Issues in Social Work Practice and Ethics in Research Practice and Innovation published by IGI Global between 2018-2019. He has published over 150 papers in scientific journals, of which 60 are WoS indexed, the author holding an H factor of 13 in WoS and an H factor of 25 in Google Scholar. He is also the author of over 20 volumes in Romanian and English.

For more information about the author ☞ ☞

SCAN ME

Thank you for reading this book!

If you have 60 seconds, hearing your honest feedback on Amazon would mean a lot to me.
It does wonders for the book, and I love hearing about your experience with it!

To leave your feedback:

1. Open your camera app
2. Point your mobile device at the **QR code** below
3. The review page will appear in your web browser

Or visit

https://www.amazon.com/dp/B0FLMDKNNZ

Thank you!

www.ingramcontent.com/pod-product-compliance
Lightning Source LLC
Chambersburg PA
CBHW071340230926
51846CB00002B/403
9789731666471